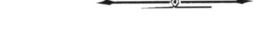

ISBN 978-0-331-09750-4
PIBN 11013733

Tuberculosis

OF

The Nose and Throat

BY

LORENZO B. LOCKARD, M. D.

LARYNGOLOGIST AND RHINOLOGIST TO THE JEWISH CONSUMPTIVES RELIEF
SOCIETY SANATORIUM, THE Y. M. C. A. HEALTH FARM AND THE EVAN-
GELICAL LUTHERAN SANATORIUM; FORMERLY LARYNGOLOGIST
TO THE NATIONAL JEWISH HOSPITAL FOR CONSUMPTIVES
AND MEMBER OF THE BOARD OF DIRECTORS OF THE
AGNES MEMORIAL SANATORIUM; ONE TIME
PROFESSOR OF ANATOMY, TOLEDO MED-
ICAL COLLEGE; FELLOW OF THE
AMERICAN ACADEMY OF
OPHTHAMOLOGY AND
OTO-LARYNGOL-
OGY, ETC.

WITH EIGHTY-FIVE ILLUSTRATIONS, SIXTY-FOUR OF THEM
IN COLORS.

C. V. MOSBY MEDICAL BOOK & PUBLISHING CO.

St. Louis,

1909

Press of
Stewart Scott Press Rooms,
St. Louis, Mo.

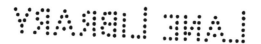

PREFACE

The annual mortality from tuberculosis, in the United States, approximates 150,000, and from eight to ten times this number are affected, to some extent, with the disease.

Statistics compiled from all parts of the world, including private as well as hospital and sanatoria records, show that complicating lesions of the throat occur in at least one-third of all persons with recognizable foci in the lungs. Autopsies upon individuals dead of consumption prove that nearly fifty per cent have tuberculous lesions in the larynx, but assuming only one of every four consumptives to be so affected, an ultra-conservative estimate, the fact is established that none other of the serious diseases to which the upper respiratory tract is subject approaches tuberculosis in prevelancy nor in the unhappy consequences which it entails.

In every case the development of a focus in the larynx or pharynx increases greatly the gravity of the constitutional malady, in many it produces prolonged, and at times, almost intolerable pain and in a considerable proportion it proves the direct cause of death. Experience has demonstrated, however, that the larger number of such infections are preventable,

40486

that at least one-half of the already developed lesions can be brought to the stage of arrest, and that in the majority of those that do not so respond the more distressing symptoms may be held in partial subjection.

The chief reasons for the high mortality that has been witnessed are to be found, first, in the almost universal neglect to make systematic examinations of the larynx in pulmonary patients until subjective symptoms have developed, by which time the lesions have often passed the bounds of incipiency and the general vitality has become hopelessly impaired, and secondly, in the generally accepted but erroneous beliefs that laryngeal tuberculosis is almost invariably fatal and that treatment commonly does more harm than good.

Early lesions subjected to treatment are usually curable, and the advanced not infrequently so, and when these facts are recognized the pessimism that rules to-day will be succeeded by a rational optimism with the natural results thereof; more persistent, prompt and intelligent, and therefore more effective management of all such cases.

The main objects of this book are to place before the profession the modern views concerning the early recognition, the treatment and prognosis of the disease, in the hope that an increased faith in the efficacy of treatment and a full appreciation of the importance of early diagnosis and of routine examinations of the larynx in every consumptive, will be engendered.

The author desires to make cordial acknowledgment of the writings of Gerber, Heymann and Wright, to which he is indebted for much of the historical and pathological material, and of all the classical works on

Laryngology and Tuberculosis, from which he has at times freely translated and quoted.

Of the drawings, Figures 2 and 3 are taken from the Seifert-Kahn Atlas, and Figure 4 from the well known work of Heinze.

All the other illustrations are the work of Fred'k L. Cavally, Jr., and, with a few exceptions, were made from specimens and patients under the direct supervision of the author, who takes this opportunity of expressing his appreication of the skill and painstaking care given by the artist to every detail of the work.

Denver, Colorado, November, 1908.

CONTENTS.

CHAPTER I.

HISTORICAL SURVEY OF LARYNGEAL TUBERCULOSIS.

CHAPTER II.

ETIOLOGY—PRIMARY AND SECONDARY INFECTIONS.

CHAPTER III.

ETIOLOGY—ENDOGENETIC AND EXOGENETIC INFECTION.

CHAPTER IV.

Etiology—Predisposing Causes.

CHAPTER V.

Pathology.

CHAPTER VI.

Subjective Symptoms.

CHAPTER VII.

Objective Symptoms.

CHAPTER VIII.

Diagnosis.

CHAPTER IX.

PROGNOSIS.

CHAPTER X.

RECORDS.

CHAPTER XI.

HYGIENIC AND DIETETIC TREATMENT.

CHAPTER XII.

MEDICINAL TREATMENT.

CHAPTER XIII.

SURGICAL TREATMENT—ENDOLARYNGEAL OPERATIONS.

CHAPTER XIV.

SURGICAL TREATMENT—EXTRALARYNGEAL OPERATIONS.

CHAPTER XV.

THE NOSE.

CHAPTER XVI.

THE NASO-PHARYNX.

CHAPTER XVII.

THE PHARYNX.

LARYNGEAL TUBERCULOSIS

CHAPTER I.

THE LARYNX.

HISTORY.

An historical survey of laryngeal tuberculosis can be most conveniently made by a division into epochs; epochs of achievement rather than the arbitrary one of years, or in other words, by considering the notable steps through which we have arrived at our present state of knowledge. These epochs are:—

1. Period antedating and including the recognition of the laryngeal tubercle, 400 B. C· to 1825 A. D.

2. First attempts at differentiation of phthisis and syphilis, 1829 to 1842.

3. Period of pathologic investigation, beginning 1842.

4. Period of clinical observation, beginning 1858.

5. Determination of the true nature of laryngeal phthisis, 1879.

6 Inauguration of a rational therapy, 1886

First Period:—The symptoms of consumption were clearly described by Hippocrates (460-377 B. C.), and as he alluded to "ulcers in the tube of the lungs," it may justly be inferred that he had some conception of the disease as it appears in the larynx.

From this time on no real advance, in so far as the larynx is concerned, was made until Matthew Baillie (The Works of Matthew Baillie, Vol. II, Page 84, 1825) described tubercles of the larynx and trachea with inflammation and ulceration of the mucosa, associated with "scrofulous abscesses of the lungs."

This description, in the posthumous edition of his "Works, 1825," shows his observations to have been made between this date and the year 1793, when in the "Morbid Anatomy of Some of the Most Important Parts of the Human Body," he referred to the frequent appearance of tubercles in the lungs, but denied their occurrence in the branches of the trachea, "where there are follicles."

That tubercules of the laryngeal mucosa were definitely recognized at this time is further evidenced by a description of white miliary tubercles in the larynx of a man dead of pulmonary phthisis, by Broussais, in the *Histoire des Phlegmasies*, 1816.

The pulmonary tubercle had been recognized and described during a period of almost two hundred years before Baillie and Broussais noted a corresponding condition of the larynx.

Thus Sylvius (1614-1672) maintained the identity of the nodules found in the lungs and the disease known as phthisis, but erroneously considered the nodules to be enlarged lymph glands. Morton, 1689, showed that the turbercle was the necessary precursor of ulceration, and somewhat later, 1700, Magnetus described miliary tubercles.

Fragmentary descriptions of various laryngeal lesions classified under the common name of phthisis, in which this disease and syphilis were hopelessly confused, were given by Morgagni (*De Sedibus et Causis Morborum*, 1762) and Lieutaud)*Histoire Anatomica Medica*, 1767).

Morgagni recorded two cases that have been commonly accepted as a definite recognition of phthisis, although there is no indisputable proof that they were not syphilitic.

The one, quoted from Fantoni, concerned a man who for a long time before death suffered from severe dyspnea. Post-mortem examination showed a larynx so constricted by infiltration and ulceration of the arytenoid cartilages that only a small aperture remained.

In 1704 Valsalva performed an autopsy upon an unmarried woman of forty who had been a long time sufferer from symptoms presumably due to asthma.

No cause for death being found, Valsalva, at Morgagni's suggestion, opened the larynx from behind. It was extensively ulcerated and filled with a crum like grayish colored pus, fully accounting for the long continued dyspnea.

Lieutaud's cases are somewhat similar and it is impossible to conjecture which of these two constitutional conditions, syphilis or phthisis, was responsible.

Lieutaud's carefulness of research, however, is shown by his description, after numerous post-mortems, of the first two cases of laryngeal polypi.

At this period phthisis was not alone confused with syphilis, but with all diseases accompanied by ulceration, swelling, necrosis and abscess formation; i. e., carcinoma, perichondritis, etc.

Petit (*Diss. de phthisie laryngea*, Montpelier, 1790);

Sauvée (*Rech. s. l. phthisie laryngée*, Paris, 1802);
Sigaud (*Rech. s. l. phthisie laryngée*, Strassb., 1819);
and Portal (*Obser. sur la Nature et sur le Traite-
ment de la Phthisie pulmonaire*, Paris, 1792), gave
fairly comprehensive descriptions of the disease without, however, differentiating the tuberculous and
syphilitic cases.

By the end of the century the science of laryngology
had only advanced to a stage permitting a division of
laryngeal diseases into three groups; phthisis, croup
and acute inflammations.

Sachse (*Beitr. z. genaueren Kenntnisz und Unter-
scheidung der Kehlkopf-u. Luftröhenschwindsuchten*,
Hanover, 1821) and three years later Pravaz (*Rech.
et observ. p. serv. à l'hist. de la phthisie laryng. Thèse
de Paris*), collected many cases and gave a complete
resumé of the literature preceding and including the
era in which they wrote.

The confusion of various diseases at this time,
however, is shown by Pravaz's statement that, "No
one can doubt to-day that laryngeal phthisis may exist
primarily."

These "primary" cases were cured by the administration of mercury.

Many theories were advanced as to the etiology of
phthisical ulcerations of the larynx, and Columbat
credited them to enlargment of the tonsils and uvula.

Louis (*Recherches Anatomica Pathologique sur la
Phthisie*, 1825) made the first real attempt at exact
study and classification and although he failed to sub-
stantiate Baillie and Broussais in regard to the occurrence of laryngeal tubercles, he noted their fre-

quent appearance in the lungs. He credited laryngeal infection to the mechanical irritation of the mucosa by the poisonous pulmonary excretions, and maintained that those points most subject to insult by the passing secretions were most frequently affected, and that therefore the danger of infection decreased proportionately to the distance of the parts from the affected pulmonary areas.

This last observation was undoubtedly based upon the records of his post-mortems on the "tracheal artery" in 102 cases of pulmonary consumption, where he found tracheal involvement 31 times, laryngeal 22, and epiglottic 18 times.

Louis's conception of etiology, while containing much of error, had a germ of truth and has been accepted to a certain degree by many modern observers.

The theory that some tuberculous ulcers are of a catarrhal nature, long maintained by him, and to which he reverts in the 1843 edition of his works, has been generally abandoned but the majority of present day investigators credit the occurrence of some lesions —the so-called arrosion, corrosion or diphtheritic ulcers—to the mechanical irritation produced by cough, cachexia and sputum, resulting in superficial necrosis and subsequent infection by the bacillus.

The existence of catarrhal ulcers in the larynges of tuberculous individuals is strongly combatted by Jonathan Wright.

Borsieri in 1826 said: "There are those who think ulcers of the larynx and the aspera arteria, because they are not situated in the lungs, should be excluded from phthisis. However, from these lesions also the

body often wastes away, and is consumed by a slow
fever just as in the parent disease.''

Second Period:—Albers (*Die Pathol. u. Therap. der
Kehlkopfkrankheiten*, Leipzig, 1829), in a painstaking
review of the literature of laryngeal phthisis, noted
the occurrence of tubercles and gave a lucid description of their clinical appearance and transformation
into ulcers.

To this author can be accredited the first serious attempt to differentiate tuberculosis and syphilis, and
this may well be considered the second great step
toward an intelligent understanding of the disease as
localized in the larynx.

A decade later, Barth (*Mémoire sur les ulcerations
des voies aeriennes, Archives Generales de Medicine*,
1839) succeeded in furthering the differential diagnosis
of the two conditions.

Three years before this communication by Barth,
Trousseau and Belloc won the prize offered by the
Paris Academy for the best difinition and description
of laryngeal phthisis, in their essay entitled: "*Traité
Prat. de la Phthisie Laryngée Chronique, et des Mala-
dies de la Voix*, 1837."

They defined the disease as "*tout altération du larynx, pouvant amener la consomption ou la mort, en
quelque maniére que ce soit.*"

They maintained the principle of occasional primary
localization of the tuberculous process in the larynx, a
much discussed question at the present time, but
admitted its general dependence upon preceding pulmonary involvement.

They included in their category of laryngeal phthisis:

"1. Simple laryngeal phthisis produced by the common causes of inflammation in general, without pulmonary phthisis.

"2. Syphilitic laryngeal phthisis.

"3. Cancerous laryngeal phthisis.

"4. Tubercular laryngeal phthisis.

"Notwithstanding their recognition of tubercle in their last division, we see in their first the influence of the catarrhal theory of Louis." Cit. from Jonathan Wright (The Nose and Throat in Medical History).

In this essay they outlined the first rational therapy for laryngeal diseases:—douches, swabbing and the auto-insufflation of powders through curved cannulae.

Third Period:—With Rokitansky we note a still further advance in the differentiation of phthisis and syphilis, and what was of infinitely greater worth in its influence upon the advancement of laryngology, a beginning of comprehensive study of the morbid lesions of tuberculous and other laryngeal diseases. While many of the ideas advanced by him were later abandoned, others were based upon truths that obtain to a considerable degree in the pathology of to-day.

In the "*Lehrbuch d. Path. Anat.*, 1842-'46," he describes the tubercle as an exudate of inspissated proteins, and states that tubercles and scrofulous glands are identical structures, and that ulcers result from the breaking down of the exudate. He likewise deals with the question of predisposition, the tuberculous habitus, and considers it of great importance.

Tubercles of the air passages frequently occur—most often in the larynx, rarely in the trachea and larger bronchi, and again more frequently in the smaller tubes.

In the larynx their favorite site is the posterior wall over the musculus transversus, an observation substantiated to-day by clinical research.

The theory that tuberculous ulcerations of the larynx are dependent upon mechanical injury through the anatomical relationship of the parts, and especially when these favored areas have been previously reduced in resistance through injury or inflammation, was advanced by Rheiner (*Ueb. d. Ulcerations proc. im Larynx*, Virch. Arch., v., 1853) and fourteen years later by Colberg (*Beitr. z. norm. u. path. Anat. d. Lunge, Arch. f. Klin. Med.*, II, 1867).

The basis of this theory was the assumption that ulcerations generally occur upon symmetrical points, points which normally come in contact during the physiologic movements of the larynx, i. e., the vocal processes in speaking and the free edge of the epiglottis and the tips of the arytenoids in swallowing. In refutation of this it is only necessary to suggest that initial lesions are rarely seen upon these "favored" points; on the epiglottis the usual location is the laryngeal surface, the tip usually becoming affected at a later period through extension, while the vocal processes are not involved to a much greater extent than the other segments of the cords.

Neither the epiglottis nor the arytenoids exhibit the same percentage of involvement as other points not subject to rubbing or pressure, i. e., the vocal cords and inter-arytenoid sulcus, and the ventricular bands are more often affected than the epiglottis.

In this period was first advanced the idea of a transference of infection in phthisis from the lungs to the larynx by way of the nerve trunks, particularly the vagus (Friedreich: *Handb. d. Spec. Path. u. Ther., Bd. V.,* 1854). This view was supported as late as 1888 by Libermann (*De l'Étiologie de la Phthisie Pulmonaire et Laryngée*).

While Friedreich totally misconceived the true basic facts of etiology, he attempted to differentiate between the tubercles in tuberculosis and the small gray nodules due to simple inflammation of the mucosa.

In the "*Handbuch d. Spec. Path. u. Ther.,* Stuttgart, 1856," Wunderlich showed the influence of Louis, and of Trousseau and Belloc, in his statement that the greater number of ulcerations occurring in the larynges of tuberculous individuals are of a purely catarrhal origin.

He recognized the rarity of true tuberculosis of the trachea, and its comparatively frequent appearance in the larynx, especially in those cases where the lung disease is of long standing and accompanied by colossal secretions.

Fourth Period:—The period of clinical study began with the demonstration of the practical utility of the laryngoscope, by the Maestro, Manuel Garcia, in 1855. (Physiol. Observ. on Human Voice.)

During the preceding half-century many attempts were made to see into the interior of the larynx by means of variously conceived cannulae, mirrors and prisms, i. e.: Bozzini, 1807; Senn, 1827; Babbington,

1828; Beaumés, 1838; Liston, 1840; Trousseau and Belloc, 1837; Warden, 1844; Türck, 1857, and Czermak, 1858.

Many of these appliances were based upon the principle afterwards adopted by Garcia, but for various reasons failed of common adoption.

Immediately following Garcia's communication the science of clinical laryngology was born and advanced with giant strides, and laryngeal phthisis, so long misunderstood and obscured by a cloud of false ideas, emerged almost at once into the light, freed from most of the old misconceptions.

The pioneer work was largely performed by C. Gerhart (Gerhardt und Roth, *Ueber Syphil. Krankheiten d. Kehlkopfes, Virch. Arch.*, 21, 1860) in detailing a large series of cases examined by the new method. In this thesis he clearly described syphilis and succeeded in finally separating it from phthisis.

This work was soon supplemented by another upon the influence of catarrhal swelling of the posterior laryngeal wall in the production of aphonia. (*Ueber einige Ursachen Katarrhal Heiserkeit, Würzburger medic. Zeitschr.*, Bd. III, 1862.)

In this essay he considered the possible influence of an apparently simple catarrh upon the development of tuberculosis, and believed that this condition might be of considerable etiologic import.

In 1861, in the "*Tr. Clin. d. mal. d. enfants*, Rilliet and Barthez," we find the first reference in regard to the influence of age. They state that ulcerations in the upper respiratory tract occur usually after the seventh year of life, and very rarely before the age of three to four years, and that while usually dependent upon advanced pulmonary disease, they may occur as a result of other organic tuberculous processes.

They agree with Louis as to etiology, and maintain the general dependence of laryngeal ulcers upon preceding advanced disease of the lungs or other organs.

To the theory of Rheiner, the mechanical injury of symmetrical points, Türck (*Klin. d. Kehlkopfkrankh., Wien*, 1866), one of the most careful observers, reverts, and concludes that this is the most frequent form, while the true tuberculous ulcers occur in but a small proportion of cases.

As late as 1872 we again find this idea of the non-tuberculous nature of many ulcerations advanced by Waldenberg (*D. loc. Behandl. d. Krankheiten d. Athmungsorgane*), who explains his conviction on the ground that many ulcers of the larynx in phthisical individuals heal completely, and are therefore merely follicular ulcerations.

The earliest descriptions of the tuberculous tumor were given by Tobold (*D. chron. Kehlkopfkrankh.*, 1866); Mandl (*Tr. prat. d. mal. d. larynx et pharynx,* Paris, 1872) and Ariza (*Anfiteatro, anat. Espanol,* 1877).

The first of these described cases in the incipient stages of laryngeal tuberculosis where the entire glottis was filled with tumors of the mucosa. The growths were pale in color, of cauliflower formation, and appeared mainly in the ventricles, on the vocal processes and the posterior wall.

Rindfleisch (*Lehrb. d. Path. Anat.*, 1873) upheld in a slightly modified way the theory of Rheiner and Türck, i. e., the irritation of symmetrical segments of the larynx by the infectious products of a scrofulous catarrh. The persistence of this idea has been shown at length, both because of its important place in history and because many more modern observers have given it a prominent place in etiology.

In studying the further progress of knowledge it is necessary to revert to the role played by the tubercle.

Lewin (*Ueb. Krankh. einz. Theile d. Larynx, etc., Virch. Archiv.* XXIV, 1862) believed some erosion of the mucosa to be an almost necessary antecedent to the deposit of tubercles, or at least that the tubercles usually develop in such damaged spots.

That the tuberculous ulcer is a result of the disintegration of tubercles he clearly recognized, and likewise the existence of small granulations about the edges of such ulcers, the first reference to this important characteristic.

Virchow (*Geschwülste,* 1864 and '65,) took strong exception to Louis's assertions regarding the mechanical cause of phthisical ulcers, and made it plain that laryngeal tuberculosis is due to the tubercle and nothing else, and reasserted the fact that ulceration is consequent upon destruction of the tubercle.

He recommended the larynx as the best locality in which to study the tubercle, which he described as follows: "In the very frequent tuberculosis of the larynx, small, flat, clear, grey or whitish swellings are found, which hardly project beyond the surface." These tubercles never caseate or form tumors.

R. Meyer (*D. gegenw. Stand. d. Fr. v. d. Kehlkopfschwindsucht. Correspondenzbl. f. Schweizer Aerzte, Nr.* 13, 1873) combatted this view of Virchow's as to the relation of the tubercle to ulcerative laryngeal phthisis, upon the ground that he had been unable to find tubercles in laryngeal ulcerations and that therefore they could play no part in its production. Ten years later Bosworth reverted to the old theory of the non-tuberculous nature of some laryngeal lesions in phthisis.

Almost coincidently with Virchow, Förster (*Lehrb. d. path. Anat.*, 1864) expressed the same views, and gave as the favorite site of the tubercles the interarytenoid sulcus, and described their ultimate conversion into crater-shaped ulcers, confluent, with sequelae of cartilage necrosis and abscess formation. He believed the tubercle might be either primary or secondary.

Bruns (*Die Laryngoskopie u. laryng. Chirurgie*, 1865) credited laryngeal ulcers to one of two sources:

1. Disease of the mucous follicles.
2. Circumscribed deposits in the submucosa (tubercles).

The dependence of epithelial necrosis upon submucous deposits was further elaborated by Tobold (*Laryngosk. u. Kehlkopfkrankh.*, 1867) who ascribed the necrosis to the gradually increasing pressure from beneath, with ultimate loosening of the mucosa from its attachment, or in some instances, to the degeneration of miliary tubercles.

From this time on advance in the knowledge of pathology was rapid and unbroken, the chief work being done by E. Wagner, Waldenburg, Rindfleisch, V. Ziemssen and Heinze.

Wagner (*D. Tuberkelähnl. Lymphadenom. Arch. f.*

Heilk., 11-12, 1870 and '71) minutely pictured the typical tuberculous infiltrate, tubercle and ulcer.

Waldenburg (*D. loc. Behandl. d. Krankh. d. Athmungsorgane,* Berlin, 1872) described the occurrence, about the edges of tuberculous ulcers, of miliary tubercles, but was uncertain as to whether they were the cause or a product of the ulcers. With many observers he agreed in considering a large proportion of laryngeal ulcers in consumptives to be purely catarrhal, a conclusion based upon the rapidity with which some of these ulcers healed.

A new view point was assumed by Sommerbrodt (*Ueb. d. Abhängigk. phthisischer Lungenerkrankh. v. prim. Kehlkopfaffectionen, Arch. f. Exper. Path. u. Pharm.,* 1873) in his contention that pulmonary phthisis might be caused by purulent peribronchitis acting through a chronically inflamed larynx and trachea.

V. Ziemssen (*Handb. d. spec. Path. u. Ther., Bd.* IV, 1, 1876) classified tuberculous laryngeal ulcerations as follows:

1.   Ulcerations due to miliary tuberculosis and tuberculous inflammations consequent upon pulmonary phthisis.

2.   Follicular ulcerations.

3.   Ulcers dependent upon specific cell infiltration.

4.   Superficial aphthous, or erosion ulcers.

He likewise maintained the usual dependence of laryngeal ulcerations upon disease of the lungs and claimed that healing, while possible, was extremely rare.

Fifth Period:—The credit of reconciling these many

conflicting conjectures belongs to Oscar Heinze, who in 1879, (*D. Kehlkopfschwindsucht,* Leipzig) demonstrated that the sole cause of laryngeal and tracheal tuberculosis is tuberculous infiltration of the mucosa, and that ulceration in the larynx and trachea never leads to tuberculosis unless there is simultaneous or subsequent tuberculosis of the mucous membranes.

This view was subscribed to by all the later investi- gators except Beverly Robinson (Ulcerative Phthisi- cal Laryngitis, *Amer. Jour. of Med. Sciences,* April, 1879) who claimed that ''the ulcerations which have been described in the larynx under the name of miliary tubercles are none other, as a rule, than small spheri- cal swellings, which are occasioned by the filling up with transparent fluid of the closed follicles of the submucous reticulum, which have been described by Heitler and Coyne.''

Heinze believed in the simultaneous existence of tuberculous and catarrhal ulcers.

Sixth Period:—The record of advancement in ther- apy is meager. Galen (129-200 A. D.) declared that ulcers of the ''arteria aspera'' were easily curable, but this impression was combatted by Marcellus Donatus (*De Historia Medica Mirabili Lib.,* 1613) and his views, in so far as they concern tuberculosis, have ob- tained until the present time.

During this entire period but few procedures were offered for relief through either surgical or medicinal agencies.

In 1818 it was suggested that some benefit followed the use of creosote in the form of tar fumigations.

Albers, in 1829, (*Die Path. u. Ther. der. Kehlkopf-krankheiten*) advocated the performance of tracheotomy and claimed for it a wonderful influence through the complete rest given the larynx.

The use of steam inhalations, swabbing, douches and the auto-insufflation of powders was advised by Trousseau and Belloc in 1837.

A year later Horace Green succeeded in making applications of silver nitrate to the interior of the larynx, by means of curved applicators similar to those in use at the present time. His report was published in 1846 under the caption: "Treatise on Diseases of the Air Passages, comprising an Inquiry into the History, Pathology, Causes and Treatment of those Affections of the Throat called Bronchitis, Chronic Laryngitis, Clergyman's Sore Throat, etc." Green's pretensions were bitterly denounced by the profession, the greater number claiming such a procedure to be absolutely impracticable. Finally, after suffering the severest of calumnies, he succeeded in proving his claims and in having the method of treatment upheld.

William Marcet (Clinical Notes on Diseases of the Larynx, London, 1869) advocated puncture of the involved tissues, but the surgical treatment received no further impetus until the resurrection of Albers' suggestion of the utility of tracheotomy, by Moritz Schmidt, in 1880 (*Die Kehlkopfschwindsucht und ihre Behandlung, Arch. f. Klin. Medicin.*, Bd. 25, 1880). In addition to tracheotomy he strongly recommended, in selected cases, the use of scarification and incision of the laryngo-pharyngeal wall.

Surgery, however, owes its present recognized position to the work of Heryng (*Beitr. z. chir. Behandl. d. tubercul. Larynxphthise. d. Med. Woch.*, 1886, and *Die Heilbarkeit der Larynx phthisie und ihre Chirurgishe Behandlung*, 1887), who advocated curettage and claimed to have effected many cures through its performance.

Two years before this, Krause (*Berlin Klin. Wochenschrift*, Nr. 26, 1885) introduced lactic acid and reported many favorable results. Consequent upon these two recommendations the pendulum swung from the extreme pessimism that had ruled from earliest times, to enthusiastic optimism, to recede once again to an illogical point when the high promises regarding the universal utility of these agents remained unfulfilled.

Lactic acid, however, is still recognized as one of the most valuable agents for combatting ulceration, and the surgical treatment has steadily gained in favorable consideration, especially upon the Continent. In America, with a few notable exceptions, it has failed to secure the endorsement it undoubtedly deserves, although at the present time there seems to be some recrudescence in its favor.

CHAPTER II.

ETIOLOGY.

The upper respiratory tract, owing to its anatomical position, relationships and conformation, exhibits in certain segments a marked susceptibility to infection by the tubercle bacillus. The results of this infection become manifest in any or all of the protean forms of the disease recognized as typical in other organs—infiltrations, granulations, ulcerations, tuberculomata, miliary tubercles and lupus.

THEORY OF PRIMARY AND SECONDARY INFECTION.

The chief contention from an etiologic standpoint concerns the route by which the tubercle bacillus, the invariable causative agent, gains entrance into the tissues.

Two theories are advanced, the one of primary infection depending upon the assumption of an initial lesion of the nose, pharynx, or larynx as the case may be, the infecting material being deposited by the ingested food or inspired air; the other assuming a primary involvement of some distant organ, usually the lungs, with an infection of the upper tract through the agency of bacilli-laden sputum, or by way of the blood or lymph vessels.

In so far as the larynx is concerned, the possibility of an occasional primary infection has apparently been proven by the post-mortem investigations of Orth, Pogrebinski and Demme, in cases where, with undoubted laryngeal tuberculosis, the lungs were found to be entirely normal.

These cases, in connection with a few others of a less definite nature, would be absolutely conclusive were it not for one factor which may invalidate previously accepted conclusions—the possibility of infection of the larynx by way of the lymphatic glands.

Latent tuberculosis of any of the constituent parts of the lymphatic system, particularly of the tonsils and bronchial glands, may exist for years without symptoms or alterations in their macroscopic images, and yet from such foci, through lymphatic or blood transmission or perhaps by direct transmission through the tissue spaces, a secondary laryngeal focus might become established, particularly if the involved gland has been subject to traumatism or to the action of such inflammatory processes a scarlet fever and measles. That such a nidus, even when situated within the the interior of the gland, may become the point of departure for other widely disseminated processes has been repeatedly demonstrated.

Cornet has seen general miliary tuberculosis follow an experimentally induced focus of small size in such a lymph gland, and various observers, notably Volland, have witnessed the invasion of the lung by bacilli from the cervical glands.

Tuberculous peritonitis has been known to have its origin in a tonsillar lesion, and Shurley, in considering this source of infection says: "Much enlarged adenoid glands at the vault of the pharynx, especially with diseased conditions of the follicles or lymph spaces, are often conducive to the accession of pulmonary diseases."

The relations of the lymphatics of the larynx to neighboring structures need not be considered for infection does not invariably follow in the direction of the lymph current; it may take a course vertical or directly opposed to it.

Upon this point Cornet writes: "Dissemination from the primary gland takes not only a centripetal, but also a radial direction, in such wise that the main movement sets in toward the heart, along with the lymph current; that minor movements take a course vertical to that of the lymph current; finally, that there is a slight tendency, often imperceptible or even entirely lacking, to spread in a direction opposed to that of the lymph current."

Invasion may also occur through the tissue spaces without leaving trace of its passage.

The frequency of this latent lymphatic condition is shown by a study of recent statistics.

In forty cadavers, thirty of which during life had shown no signs of tuberculosis, Pizzini found latent disease of the bronchial glands in 42 per cent.

Cornet found the same conditions in four, and Spengler in six children who had died of diphtheria, sepsis and peritonitis.

Jackson (*Boston Med. and Surg. Journal*, May 12, '04) reported the following:

18 cases—Tuberculous meningitis.
1 case —No history obtainable.
2 cases—Tuberculosis found on general examination.
14 cases—No history of tuberculosis.

AUTOPSIES.

16 cases—Evidence of chronic tuberculosis.
9 cases—Pulmonary tuberculosis.
7 cases—Tuberculous bronchial glands.

Demme claims that these glands, i. e., the bronchial, are diseased in 80 per cent of all cadavers, and Neumann found them involved eight times in 105 autopsies upon children supposedly non-tuberculous.

Examinations of the tonsils show equally surprising results. In studies made of apparently healthy or hypertrophied tonsils, from subjects not known to have had tuberculosis, the following results were tabulated:

AUTHOR.	Cases.	Tonsillar Involvement: Pharyngeal and Faucial.
Lermoyez	32	2
Gottstein	33	4
Brindel	64	8
Lartigan and Nicoll	75	12
Wright	63	0
Pluder & Fischer	32	5
Pilliet	10	3
Broca	100	0
Dieulafoy	61	8
Dieulafoy	35	7
Ruge	18	6
McBride & Turner	100	3
Cornil	70	4
Dempel	15	1
Piffl	100	3
Lewin	200	10
Schreiber	29	2
Hynitsche	180	7
Friedmann	145	6
Tarchetti & Zanconi	17	0
Baup	45	1
Ito	10	0
Rethi	100	6
Maccayden & MacConkey	78	0
Wex	210	7
Theissen	45	2
Lathan	45	7
Lockard	74	5
	1,986	119=5.9%

In tuberculosis of the cervical glands it is estimated that 90 per cent of the infections originate in the tonsils.

Friedmann makes the following tabulation of 91 tonsils examined post-mortem, taken (with one exception) from subjects under five years of age:

1 tonsil - - -	Riddled with tubercles. Bacilli present in large numbers. No other lesions in body.
4, and probably 5 other cases -	Tonsillar tuberculosis probably primary. Partly complicated by secondary involvement of glands, intestines and bones.
7 other cases -	Giant cells but no bacilli.
2 other cases -	Tuberculosis present, but not primary.
3 other cases -	Giant cells, but condition not tuberculous.
8 cases - - -	General tuberculosis without tonsillar. Old scars in tonsils, the result of early tuberculosis.
2 other cases -	Similar but less distinctive results.
4 cases - - -	Internal without tonsillar tuberculosis.
3 cases - - -	Bacilli found in smears from surface of tonsils, but no tuberculous changes found.

Baup, in 841 cases, including 48 of his own, found 53, or 6 per cent, tuberculous.

Rethi found bacilli present in six of 100 hypertrophied tonsils removed from persons showing no signs of tuberculosis.

Walsham, in 34 autopsies on patients dead of tuberculosis, found the tonsils tuberculous in 20.

Bâbes, in the Children's Hospital at Budapest, discovered tuberculosis of the lymph glands, particularly of the mediastinum and bronchi, in more than one-half of the autopsies.

Strassmann, in 21 autopsies upon phthisical subjects, demonstrated tonsillar involvement in 13.

The author, in 74 tonsils from subjects showing no signs of tuberculosis, found five tuberculous. The removal of one of these was followed by the accession of the disease in the cervical lymphatics and larynx.

From an examination of the tonsils of 200 subjects, L. Lewin makes the following deductions:

> 1. Hyperplastic pharyngeal tonsils conceal tuberculous lesions in about 5% of the cases.
>
> 2. The tuberculosis is present in the so-called tumor form, and is characterized by the absence of surface indications of its presence.
>
> 3. This latent tuberculosis may apparently be the first and, indeed, the only localization of the disease in the individual.
>
> 4. It is generally, however, associated with other tuberculous processes, generally of the lungs, which may, however, not have developed at the time the tonsil was operated upon.
>
> 5. It is a comparatively frequent condition among those suffering from tuberculosis of the lungs.
>
> 6. It is found in the normal-sized tonsil as well as the hyperplastic.

These few cases previously cited (*Orth, Demme, Pogrebinski*), culled from the entire voluminous literature and quoted by all authors as the most typical upon which to base the claim of occasional primary localization of the tuberculous process in the larynx, cannot therefore be accepted as definitely establishing the supposition without further confirmatory evidence, for not only must lesions of the lungs be excluded but of the lymphatic system as well. In the above cited cases no cognizance was taken of this condition. Neither is this evidence, i. e., absence of lymphatic as well as of pulmonary involvement, afforded by other reported instances.

M. Schmidt says: "I have myself seen a number of such cases of primary involvement, especially in the form of tumors of the ventricular bands and cords, but also as ulcerations." Yet none of these cases were substantiated by post-mortem examination.

Numerous other observers, among whom may be mentioned Dehio, Neidert, Fischer, Cadier and Gleitsmann, have maintained the principle of primary inoculation, based upon the observation of patients where no pulmonary lesion was manifest or in whom it developed only late in the course of the laryngeal disease. This last author, after citing two cases of cured laryngeal tuberculosis where involvement of the lungs was never clinically demonstrated, makes the admission that: "Obviously, if the postulate is brought forth that nowhere in the lungs the smallest tuberculous area exists, then the occurrence of primary laryngeal tuberculosis cannot be any longer maintained, neither in the dead nor much less in the living. But, for my part, I do not see the rationale of the argument to demand the abstract absence of the disease, in this instance of the lung, to be able to believe in the existence of another, viz., primary laryngeal tuberculosis."

It is here we have the crux of the question. Is primary infection capable of proof when other foci exist?

Central lesions of the lung, old partially cicatrized areas and new cheesy deposits in the lymph glands, bones, kidneys or retroperitoneal tissues, frequently escape the most careful search and cannot be demonstrated except upon the cadaver, yet such lesions may develop, remain unrecognized, give rise to other infections and cicatrize, or later, under fortuitous circumstances, recur.

The frequency of such lesions of the lungs has been shown by Birch-Hirschfeld:

Autopsies, 3,067; Pulmonary Tuberculosis, 41.86%; Tuberculosis cause of death, 23.3%; Old Cicatrized Pulmonary lesions, 11.97%; very early lesions, 2.8%.

When cicatrization has occurred the age of the lesion cannot be definitely ascertained, and upon this ground we must refuse to accept the evidence of such cases as those quoted by Trifiletti and Josephsohn.

The former reported the case of a girl of twenty-one years with tuberculous infiltration of the laryngeal mucosa and apparently healthy lungs, who eight months later showed the first signs of pulmonary involvement.

In Josephsohn's case the evidence of lung involvement arose two years after laryngeal phthisis was diagnosed. Similar and equally indefinite cases are reported by Ziemssen, Barth, Haslund, Garre and Moritz.

Bernheim refers to twenty-nine cases of primary laryngeal disease seen by him, without post-mortem confirmation. That such a large number of apparently primary cases should be seen by one observer is remarkable when we consider the paucity of cases from all other sources.

J. Horne has not once in ten years met with an example in the necropsies of nine large hospitals.

In 904 consecutive cases for which exact records are

available, the author has met but three in which the lung examination proved negative and in one of these the necropsy revealed a healed lesion. In a second case, one of slight laryngeal involvement in which death could not be attributed to the tuberculous process, the lungs were normal but the faucial tonsils were affected, showing the possible dependence of some laryngeal cases upon old lymphatic lesions. The third case could not be subjected to autopsy.

An oft-quoted case is that of Champeaux's, where a tumor was present on the ventricular band, with apical dullness, but no bacilli in the sputum. That such a case is absolutely without value in this connection goes without saying.

Sheedy (*Post Graduate,* XVIII, p. 164) reports a case in which the larynx was involved for nine months, with bacilli in the sputum, before the lungs became affected.

Kelson (*Laryngoscope,* April, 1903) presented before the Laryngological Society of London a man with swelling of the epiglottis, ary-epiglottic folds, ventricular bands and vocal cords, but no bacilli in the sputum.

To establish proof of this supposition, i. e., the possibility of involvement of the larynx by way of the lymphatics or blood vessels from the lymph glands, or by direct transmission through the tissue spaces, the following facts and somewhat parallel cases are adduced:

"Caries of the processus mastoideus and of the petrous bone are mostly referable to tuberculous disease of the middle ear through the lymphatic channels. A bony focus originated through infection by way of the pharyngeal tonsils."—Ruge.

"In an infection proceeding by way of the vascular system, it is of course immaterial where the primary focus is situated:"—Cornet.

In 67 autopsies (König-Orth) lesions of the bones or joints were found to be dependent upon other lesions in 53 cases—79 per cent. Of these the lungs were responsible in 37 cases, the glands in 21.

Ph. Schech reports the case of a man who in his sixty-third year had the right testicle removed because of tuberculous involvement. He remained free from the disease for two years, when the posterior pharyngeal wall became affected; then the larynx, and finally the lungs succumbed.

Another example given by the same author concerns a man who in his twenty-eighth year developed tuberculosis in the left apex with hemoptysis. After fifteen years of seemingly perfect recovery he suddenly developed tuberculosis of the ear, velum and lips.

"Laryngeal tuberculosis may be caused by lymphatic transmission from a neighboring focus, i. e., in the palate, fauces or tonsils."—Cornet.

Chiari and Riehl examined 68 persons who suffered from lupus either of the face or of the mucous membranes, but gave no subjective symptoms of laryngeal disease, and discovered lupus of the larynx in six cases.

It has been proven that a tuberculous process of the larynx itself becomes a source of further infection, either by contact, as of symmetrical portions of the larynx, or by lymphatic extension to neighboring organs, either of the mouth or pharynx. If mouth infection can result by lymphatic transmission from the larynx the converse must likewise be true, as infection occurs not only in the direction of the lymph current but in a direction directly opposed or vertical to it.

In a number of instances a retrograde infection—of the tonsils from diseased cervical glands—has been demonstrated to have taken place.

Grünwald (*Diseases of the Larynx,* 1900) remarks: "There is no doubt that diseased cervical glands are capable of infecting the larynx; many a so-called 'primary' case is no doubt due to this cause."

Two cases proving connection between disease of the larynx, cervical glands and tonsils, occurring in the author's practice, may be adduced:

Girl, *aet.* 11. Hypertrophied tonsils and small mass of adenoids. Bilateral enlargement of the cervical glands. Lungs normal and general condition good. Three months following the removal of the adenoids and tonsils, the cervical glands having in the meantime partially disappeared, hoarseness developed and examination revealed incipient tuberculosis of the left side of the larynx. The left cord was infiltrated throughout its entire extent and there was moderate infiltration of the inter-arytenoid sulcus. The further history substantiated the diagnosis, but pulmonary tuberculosis was never demonstrated. In this case we had an undoubted infection of the cervical glands from the tonsils, and of the larynx by way of the cervical glands. Examination of the tonsils had proved . them tuberculous.

The second case concerns a girl of seven years, who

had a large mass of suppurating cervical glands on the right extending from the angle of the jaw to the clavicle. The immediate cause of the consultation, however, was a retro-pharyngeal abscess of three days' duration. The tonsils were not large, but ragged, with numerous deep crypts filled with cheesy concretions. The lungs and other organs were apparently normal. The retro-pharyngeal abscess was opened, draining almost completely the mass of suppurating cervical glands. Ten days later these glands were removed and two weeks later the tonsils were completely extirpated, and on microscopic examination showed undoubted tuberculosis. At this time the first complete laryngeal examination was made, the child having previously rebelled. There was rugous infiltration of the interarytenoid sulcus, with a small ulcer at the point of union of the arytenoid cartilage, vocal cord and right ventricular band. Seven months later the child died and examination showed the lungs to be normal and the larynx tuberculous.

This case is of special interest from another standpoint; the cervical suppuration antedated the pus formation in the retro-pharynx, burrowed its way into that space, and was partially emptied through the pharyngeal incision.

McKinney (*Journal of Tuberculosis,* January, 1903) reports a case of laryngeal tuberculosis secondary to tuberculous cervical glands, and it is the generally accepted belief that in the great majority of the cases of pulmonary tuberculosis occurring in children, infection takes place from the lymph nodes; the latter may be infected in many ways. There is no certain relation between the points of entrance of the infection and the points of development of the disease.

Lartigan and Nicholl (*American Journal Medical Sciences*, June, 1902) after long research, concluded that primary tuberculosis of the pharyngeal tonsils is probably more common than is generally supposed in the production of either localized or general infection.

Upon this subject Cornet says: "Since the assumption of a primary disease, i. e., of the larynx, depends very largely upon the absence of demonstrable signs of disease in the other organs, especially the lungs, *intra vitam,* we should be very guarded, in view of the imperfections of our methods of clinical research, in inferring the primary nature of the disease."

As proving the uncertainty of the source of infection he refers to a case, classified as primary pharyngeal, reported by Isambert, of a boy of four and a half years who had tuberculous ulceration of the velum without signs of pulmonary involvement. He had, however, in early infancy shown signs of scrofula and "scrofulous (?) coryza."

Pulmonary phthisis frequently develops from disease of the cervical glands; the glands, in the majority of instances, owe their infection to previous disease of the tonsils and doubt no longer exists as to the occasional spread of the process from the cervical glands, and probably from the bronchial glands as well, to the larynx.

In view of the above proven facts, these frequently cited cases of Orth, Pogrebinski, Demme and others, can no longer be held to indisputably prove the occurrence of primary tuberculous infections of the larynx.

The probability of a direct infection of the larynx from without is extremely doubtful, although upon purely theoretical grounds the possibility must be admitted.

While the bacilli-laden air in its passage through the nose and naso-pharynx is freed from the greater number of contained organisms and dust, a small proportion penetrates into the larynx and bronchial tubes. The larger part of those introduced in this manner, and not passing onward into the lungs, is immediately expelled by the upward motion of the cilia that exist everywhere in the larynx except upon the vocal cords and posterior wall. At these points the dust particles to which the bacilli are generally attached cause an increase in the normal secretions which aid in the expulsion. When, however, owing to previous inflammations of the mucosa, erosions exist, the reflex irritability is abnormally low and many of the organisms may be retained and gain entrance through these breaks in continuity. The abraded condition of the mucosa is not always essential as it has been demonstrated that the bacilli may penetrate intact membranes, or even pass through the ducts of glands, as will be shown in discussing the etiologic role of the sputum.

If infection by inhalation plays an important role in etiology as many observers would have us believe, would it not be natural to conclude that laryngitis would occur in a larger proportion of those people who live under unhygienic surroundings and follow unhealthful occupations, than of those not subject to these disadvantages? A statistical study of these patients, however, shows that the relative proportion of laryngeal to pulmonary cases is no larger in the so-called unhealthful than in the favorable avocations, and that the same proportion maintains between individuals living in the rural communities and in the congested areas of the large cities.

If laryngeal tuberculosis occurred as a primary infection there would undoubtedly be more positive evidence in its support. When but a few cases can be adduced from such voluminous reports as are now accessible, and these take into account the condition of the lungs only, it practically removes the question beyond the pale of serious consideration. It is the almost universally accepted dictum that an absence of pulmonary foci establishes the primary nature of any existing laryngeal infection, whether or not there are foci present in other organs, but such a conclusion is absolutely unwarranted. Thus, in referring to primary laryngeal tuberculosis, Richard Lake says:

"As already mentioned, the author has seen two cases in which the larynx became affected secondarily to an apparently primary tuberculous otitis media, and in which the signs of the disease in the lungs did not show themselves until considerably later."—*Laryngeal Phthisis*, p. 93.

These cases he classified as "primary laryngeal."

A somewhat parallel case, classed as primary laryngeal tuberculosis, in which a child of four and a half years, dead of tuberculous meningitis, was found to have a laryngeal ulcer containing bacilli, is recorded by Demme.

From a purely practical standpoint, that is from a

prognostic and therapeutic point of view, a tuberculous lesion of the larynx may be considered primary when there is no demonstrable evidence of pulmonary or other organic involvement, but while theoretical considerations point to the possibility, and even the probability of such an occurrence (for there is no special peculiarity of the laryngeal mucosa or secretions to prevent it from becoming infected) we have as yet no indisputable evidence to establish it as an abstract fact.

RESUME.

1. The absence of pulmonary disease alone does not establish the primary nature of tuberculous laryngeal disease.

2. Lymphatic involvement, especially of the tonsils and cervical glands, must likewise be excluded.

3. The tonsils are tuberculous in perhaps five per cent of the cases in which hypertrophy exists.

4. It is found in the normal-sized tonsils as well as in the hyperplastic.

5. The dependence of some laryngeal cases upon disease of the tonsils and cervical glands has been clinically demonstrated.

6. Infection of the lymphatics usually follows in the direction of the lymph current, but may spread in a direction opposite, or vertical to it.

7. It may also travel through the tissue spaces.

8. But a few cases are recorded, substantiated by post-mortem investigations, in which, with lesions of the larynx the lungs have been found normal, and in these instances no reference is made to the condition of the lymphatic system.

9. There is no inherent peculiarity of the laryngeal mucosa or its secretions to prevent it from becoming primarily infected.

10. This occurrence, however, has not been demonstrated, despite the fact that phthisis is the most common and widespread of all serious laryngeal diseases.

11. From a practical standpoint, a case may be considered primary if there is no demonstrable disease of the lungs.

12. Until a case of laryngeal phthisis, unaccompanied by either pulmonary or lymphatic disease, has been proven, the assumption of primary infection cannot be maintained.

CHAPTER III.

ENDOGENETIC AND EXOGENETIC INFECTION.

While the usual and probably sole form of laryngeal phthisis has been shown to be the secondary one, opinions as to whether infection can be attributed to the direct effect of bacilli-laden sputa or to hematogenous and lymphatic deposit, diverge as widely as upon the primary question. The majority of morbid anatomists look upon sputal infection as the predominant cause, while the clinicians, with few exceptions, consider the blood and lymphatic vessels to be largely responsible. Neither school claims that the cause advocated by it is the exclusive one and thus it becomes a question of determining which factor is active in the greater number of instances. The entire domain of laryngology presents no problem of greater complexity, for almost every fact adduced in favor of one or the other theory is subject to various interpretations.

In support of the theory of infection by hematogenous or lymphatic deposit we have the fact that the laryngeal process is usually most marked upon the side where the pulmonary disease is farthest advanced, or in unilateral pulmonary involvement, the laryngeal infection is in the majority of instances upon the corresponding side. Many observers, however, have denied this localization, thus Jurasz (*Krankheiten der oberen Luftwege*) found only 7.9 per cent of 378 cases which were unilateral and corresponding.

Walsham (*Channels of Infection in Tuberculosis*) denies the frequent occurrence of lateralization, and Magenau (*Archiv. für Laryngologie, Bd.* IX, 1899) in 400 cases, found but 85 that were unilateral, and of these only 26, or 40 per cent, corresponded to the involved lung.

On the other side there is the authority of such observers as Schrötter, Schech, Friedreich, Shäffer and Krieg.

Krieg (*Archiv. für Laryngologie*, Bd. VIII, 1898) in 700 cases, found that in 275 the disease was unilateral, and in 252 of these, or 91.6 per cent, the pulmonary and laryngeal lesions were upon corresponding sides.

In 114 cases at the Agnes Memorial Sanatorium, there were 31 of unilateral laryngeal involvement, and of these 22, or 70 per cent, corresponded to the side of greater pulmonary involvement.

The author, in 904 cases, met with the following:

Laryngeal lesions unilateral in 203 cases, of which 139, or 68.4 per cent, corresponded to the pulmonary disease.

In 207 additional cases the greater involvement was upon that side where the pulmonary process was most advanced.

To offset this strong evidence of endogenetic infection, two explanations have been offered as to its probable cause:

(1)   As the primary symptom of a developing tuberculous laryngitis, before other demonstrable laryngeal or pulmonary symptoms have developed, there has occasionally been observed a unilateral paresis of the cords with intermittent hoarseness. This has been followed by other signs of local infection and finally by the appearance of pulmonary symptoms.

Schäffer reports having fond this paresis, after long observation and careful search, in 74 of 110 cases, a percentage of 67. The phenomenon has been explained by the assumption of incipient tubercles of the apex, not clinically demonstrable, pressing upon the recurrent nerve or to like action upon the part of enlarged bronchial and tracheal glands.

E. Fränkel (*Virch. Arch.*, LXXI, p. 261) attributes it in some cases to atrophy of the muscular fibres, with waxy or fatty degeneration. In some instances it may be due to an inflammatory process in the nerves themselves, the so-called "tubercular pseudo-neuroma."

The paretic condition results in loss of tone in the corresponding half of the larynx, resultant stagnation of the secretions and increased susceptibility on the part of the mucosa to infection by the sputum.

While this cause may be active in a small proportion of the cases it does not occur with sufficient frequency to invalidate the claim of an endogenetic source in the majority of instances, for apart from Schäffer, few laryngologists have witnessed it save as a rare phenomenon. The author has seen it in less than five per cent of his cases in which unilateral involvement of corresponding sides developed.

(2) It has been assumed that the entire side of the body upon which the lung infection originates is constitutionally predisposed and weakened, and that therefore the corresponding side of the larynx is first invaded.

The histologic findings have generally been interpreted as proving infection from within, i. e., by way of the blood or lymph vessels.

The first macroscopic alterations in cases of laryngeal tuberculosis are points of more or less circumscribed swelling covered by healthy mucous membrane. Histologically these swellings are found to be subepithelial tubercles, the epithelium itself and an intervening zone of varying thickness remaining entirely normal.

The distribution of the bacilli corresponds closely to the arrangement of the infiltrated tissues, decreasing in number from within out and entirely disappearing as the epithelial layer is reached.

The subepithelial distribution of the tubercles and bacilli, while strong corroborative evidence of endogenetic infection cannot be accepted as conclusive proof, for it has been experimentally proven that the bacilli can penetrate normal mucous membranes and even lymph glands without leaving trace of their entrance or passage.

The bacilli, having reached the subepithelial layers, would naturally multiply with great rapidity and thus lead to the conclusion that they had been deposited from within, as was done by Korkunoff (*D. Arch. f.*

Klin. Med., Bd. XLV) Heinze (*Kehlkopfschwindsucht,* Leipzig) and others.

Various feeding experiments in animals have shown that the bacilli may penetrate the walls of the gut, and even the skin does not offer an impenetrable barrier for its inunction with infected sputum has been followed by various tuberculous changes.

Jonathan Wright, of Brooklyn, in a drawing of a section, has shown in clearest manner the passage of bacilli through the intact epithelium.

The subepithelial distribution of the tubercle bacilli, according to E. Fränkel, is not typical. In an examination of sixteen tuberculous larynges he found as many bacilli upon the epithelial surface as within the center of the ulcer, and from this argued invasion by way of the epithelium.

The majority of his observations were made upon ulcerative cases and therefore have little weight, for they concern those cases either admittedly due to contact infection—the so-called "arrosion". ulcers—or subepithelial tubercles that through growth and degeneration have destroyed the epithelial layers with superficial spreading of the bacilli.

Moreover, of eighteen cases examined, fourteen showed streptococci and staphylococci, and he states that he invariably "found tubercle bacilli in deeper layers of the tissue than the pyogenic germs," showing conclusively, despite his former negation, that the tubercle bacilli are found chiefly below the epithelial surface.

The strongest proofs concerning the infective role of the sputum are afforded by two well-known phenomena; the localization of the infected areas and the occurrence of the so-called "arrosion," corrosion, or diphtheritic ulcers.

(1) The fact is easily demonstrable that the segments of the larynx most commonly affected are those most subject to irritation by the passing secretions. The following table shows the comparative frequency with which the various areas are involved, although some slight discrepancies will be noted in the reports of the different observers:

	Gaul	Mackenzie	Lake	Lockard	Phipps Inst.	Total
Vocal Cords	53	230	221	450	43	997
Posterior Wall.....	36	196	174	640	35	1,081
Arytenoid Cartilages	17	449	168	270	36	940
Ventricular Bands..	5	113	176	169	22	485
Epiglottis	27	186	82	127	14	436
Subglottic Space...	2	...	38	15	..	55
Total	140	1,174	859	1,671	150	3,994

From this large series of cases it is seen that the regions most frequently involved are the vocal cords, the posterior wall and the arytenoid cartilages.

The vocal cords, owing to their exposed position and to the absence of ciliated epithelium, are almost constantly bathed with the tenacious pulmonary secretions, while the points at which the sputum meets the most resistance during expulsion are the arytenoid commissure, the posterior insertion of the cords and the inner surfaces of the arytenoid cartilages.

As a general rule it may be said that infection occurs proportionately to the exposed position of the parts, but we meet with a striking exception in the case of the epiglottis.

In a total of 3,994 lesions, but 436 occurred upon the epiglottis and yet no segment of the larynx is more exposed to insult by the passing secretions, or more prone to destruction when invaded.

Several strong objections to accepting this localization as a proof of sputal infection may be advanced:

Cases of laryngeal tuberculosis are frequently seen in which the lung lesion is either quiescent or incipient, with little or no sputum and therefore practically no chance of contact infection; and conversely, many cases of advanced phthisis run their lethal course attended by colossal secretions rich in bacilli without the slightest sign of laryngeal involvement, even when local predisposition, points of *locus minoris resistentiae,* exist.

A third objection is noted in the fact that those portions of the larynx that are covered by squamous epithelium are especially subject to attack, and yet corresponding parts of the pharynx, the deep posterior and lateral walls, are rarely involved. These immune sections are natural reservoirs in which the sputum is collected and retained for much longer periods than is the case with the larynx, where reflex cough is soon called into play to aid in its expulsion.

The pharyngeal immunity may possibly be due to the fact that it is kept in a state of almost constant excitation through the passage of food and mucus, and that therefore the bacilli find little chance of lodgement, although at night these disadvantages are removed and the pharynx is as much at rest as the lower segments.

(2) *Arrosion Ulcers.*

The chief support afforded the followers of the exogenetic hypothesis is furnished by the occurrence of the so-called "arrosion" ulcers, due undoubtedly to the action of the secretions upon a normal or abraded mucosa, resulting in local necrosis and, as a general thing, subsequent infection by the tubercle bacillus.

The clearest exposition of this view has been given by Orth (*Lehrbuch der spec. path. Anat.*) who writes:

"When we have to deal with a typical case, where, perhaps, there is only a large ulcerated cavity in one apex; where all the bronchi through which the secretions from this cavity must pass during expectoration are full of tubercular ulcers; where we find smaller ulcers only on that side of the main bronchus and lower portion of the trachea, which, from the position of the body, must come into contact with the secretion, and the ulcers are found to increase in size and frequency as we ascend; where, omitting a part of the trachea, the tubercular affection is seen to be more extensive wherever the walls of the air passages are approximated and the sputum is therefore forced against the sides,—the conclusion seems inevitable that the sputum constitutes the vehicle by which the tubercular toxin is conveyed from the cavity and deposited during its transit through the air passages on favorable regions of the mucous membranes."

That infection does occur in this manner must be admitted, but as the ulcers resulting from this form of infection are relatively rare and essentially different both anatomically and clinically from the true tuberculous ulcer, which is due to the sloughing of the superficial membranes through the pressure of the constantly increasing subepithelial tubercles, their occurrence cannot militate against the theory of usual infec-

tiontion from within. The arrosion ulcers are not the
result of infiltration but are due to the degeneration
of superficial miliary tubercles. They are always superficial, have a decided tendency to spread and
fail to show, upon the floor and about the edges, the
characteristic granulations of the typical ulcers.

The base is commonly covered by a thick, yellowish
exudate that frequently forms a true fibrinous membrane elevated above the surrounding parts, hence the
older name of diphtheritic, or aphthous ulcers.

They are to be looked upon as a specific manifestation of the tuberculous process, due to contact infection, and while practically always tuberculous, they
may in occasional instances be purely catarrhal.

That is, in the larynges of tuberculous patients we
sometimes meet with small points of necrosis due to
irritation by the sputum and cough,—the same as we
sometimes have small corrosion ulcers in the vagina
or in pure catarrhal laryngitis,—but infection almost
immediately follows, hence there is small opportunity
for their observation.

Against the theory of endogenetic infection it has
been advanced that if invasion occurred through these
channels, the entire region supplied by the vessel or
vessels in fault would be equally exposed to danger,
instead of isolated parts thereof. Such a conclusion is
unwarranted; the spots where the sputum impinges
and those most irritated by cough or physiologic movements, are necessarily points of lowered resistance,
and as some previous weakening of the tissue resistance is essential to the development of tuberculous
changes, no matter in what way the toxin is conveyed,

it is at these points that infection would follow even from a widely distributed lymphatic or hematogenous deposit.

According to Cornet the assumption of a predisposition does not help the case, for he claims the more favored areas lose their apparent immunity as soon as a focus develops in their immediate neighborhood, so that they then become as liable to invasion and as little resistant to destruction when involved, as the more predisposed areas.

Although he denies that local predisposition of the larynx exists, he explains the infrequency of pharyngeal infection, in those parts unduly exposed to sputal irritation, by the assumption of some inherent property of self-defense.

Auto-infection is occasionally observable, particularly in the case of ulcers upon the edges of the cords, and supports, in very small measure, the theory of sputal infection.

As a final argument in favor of lymphatic transmission we may advance the infrequency of primary laryngeal infection.

It has been shown that in no case of tuberculous laryngitis so far studied has there been proven an absence of foci in the glands, even when the lungs were entirely free of disease. If infection occurred generally by contact, through the bacilli entering the tissues by way of gland ducts and intact epithelium, is it not reasonable to suppose, in view of the ubiquity of the bacillus, that primary laryngeal infection would be more frequently observed? Moreover, the larynx offers an exceptionally favorable point of attack, because in a large percentage of people some catarrhal inflammation, leading to points of *locus minoris resistentiae*, exists.

The connection between laryngeal and lymphatic disease in some cases has been established, and not alone of the cervical glands and tonsils but of the bronchial glands as well.

Careful consideration of all these conflicting theories which cannot be fully reconciled, permits of no other deduction than that both agencies are at fault, but that the more common route of infection is that of the blood and lymph vessels, while the role of the sputum is a not infrequent but somewhat subsidiary one.

CHAPTER IV.

PREDISPOSING CAUSES.
FREQUENCY.

Statistics bearing upon the frequency with which laryngeal phthisis occurs in consumptives vary to a striking degree:

	Pulmonary Cases	Laryngeal Involvement	Percentage
Kruse	742	123	16.6
Gaul	424	113	25.7
Eichorst (autopsies)	462	130	28.1
Heinze (autopsies)	1,226	376	30.6
De Lamallerie	502	222	44.2
Willigk	Not given	Not given	13.8
Buhl	" "	" "	15.5
Krieg	" "	" "	26.0
Frey	" "	" "	26.1
Frommel	" "	" "	40.0
Mackenzie	" "	" "	33.7
Lublinski	" "	" "	60.0
Schäffer	" "	" "	97.0
Lake, Mackenzie & Magenau	1,189	373	30.18
			34.54%

Thus the average of fourteen reports from various sections of the world is 34.5 per cent, which may be accepted as a fair estimate, although the inclusion of incipient cases through the medium of systematic examinations of all phthisical subjects, without awaiting the development of symptoms referable to the throat, would without question materially increase this percentage. A lamentable tendency to neglect routine laryngoscopic examinations exists even in many of the most up-to-date sanatoria, thus accounting in large measure for the popular misconception which regards laryngitis as a relatively uncommon complication.

The lowest percentage recorded is by Maurice Perrin (*Rev. hebd. de Laryngologie, d'Otologie,* 1902) who in 325 cases of pulmonary tuberculosis found but 1.2 per cent with laryngeal involvement.

The majority of the sanatoria refuse to admit patients with advanced laryngeal lesions and in consequence the percentage of these cases, based upon such records, is often artificially low.

Kidd (*Albutt's "System of Medicine"*) finds that 50 per cent of all cases dying of phthisis show, upon post-mortem, some tuberculous changes in the larynx.

AGE.

The age of the individual exercises a strong determining influence, and a study of the statistics shows that it is most common between the twentieth and fortieth years.

Moritz Schmidt finds that two-thirds of all the cases occur between the ages of twenty and forty.

Schrötter places the average age at thirty; Kruse from twenty to thirty; Jurasz, thirty to forty, and Heinze and Mackenzie from twenty to thirty.

In the author's cases the average has tended toward the lower limit of the above period, but some allowance must be made in considering this series, owing to the fact that it includes many cases from the Y. M. C. A. Health Farm, where most of the patients are young men in the early twenties.

The tendency of the disease to attack people between their twentieth and fortieth years is shown in the following analysis of 2,469 cases:

Age	Agnes Memorial Sanatorium	Mac-kenzie	Magenau	Lake	Author	Total
1-10	*	0	1	3	2	6
11-20	6	35	24	100	131	296
21-30	82	194	139	252	465	1,132
31-40	33	162	141	165	203	704
41-50	11	82	67	64	71	295
51 and upwards..	1	27	28	21	32	109
Totals	133	500	400	605	904	2,542

*Not admitted under 16 years.

A table by Lake shows how the proportion of consumptives attacked by tuberculous laryngitis increases up to this age period and then steadily declines:

Age	Pulmonary Phthisis	Laryngeal Ulceration	Percentage of Laryngeal Cases
Under 1 year	13	1	7.7
1-10	39	4	10.25
11-20	92	23	25.0
21-30	406	130	32.0
31-40	303	112	36.96
41-50	179	67	37.43
51-60	104	27	25.96
61-70	53	9	17.17

Wide extremes are occasionally met: Santvoord saw undoubted tuberculosis in the larynx of a child of 31 months, Schmidt in one of twelve months, and Rheindorff (*Ueb. Kehlkopftubercul. i. Kindesalter, i. Anschl. a. e. Fall v. Pseudoparalyse u. Tuberculose, Diss., Würzburg,* 1891) a case of combined tuberculosis and syphilis in a child of 13 months.

I have seen one fatal case in a child of sixteen months.

J. Solis Cohen (*American Journal of the Medical Sciences,* January, 1883) reports a case of miliary tubercles in a child of seven years.

Heinze places the percentage of laryngeal involvements occurring in infants at from two to three, and Frobelius at from two to four per cent.

Schech has seen but one case under ten years of age. Tuberculous laryngitis in children under ten years is clinically rare although it is undoubtedly more common than statistics indicate. This is due in large measure to the general impracticability of conducting thorough laryngoscopic examinations in the very young and hence the overlooking of many incipient cases.

The comparative immunity enjoyed by children may be credited in part to the fact that pulmonary consumption runs a rapid course in the young, and that a fatal termination ensues before there is time for, or a likelihood of general infection, and to the additional safeguard of an absence of preceding laryngeal disease.

The condition is rarely met with in those of advanced age but few cases having been seen after the seventieth year. The oldest of whom I have record originated in the seventy-fourth year. This case recovered. Hardie (*Laryngoscope,* July, 1905) reports a case in a man of 76, with ulceration of the epiglottis and posterior wall.

SEX.

The following table shows the relative frequency with which the two sexes are affected:

Author	No. of Cases	PROPORTION Males	Females
Mackenzie	500	2.7	1
Schmidt	2,156	2 45	1
Heinze	376	1 8	1
Kruse	...	3	1
Jurasz	...	3	1
Rosenberg	...	2	1
Lublinski	...	2	1
Magenau	400	2 7	1
Lake	667	2 8	1
Bezold	...	2	1
Phipps Institute	67	2	1
Agnes Memorial Sanatorium	133	1 9	1
Author	904	1	1
Average		2 09	1

The disparity in the proportion of the two sexes has been much less in my series than in the others reported, excepting that of the Agnes Memorial Sanatorium, and this despite the fact that cases have been included from one institution limited to male patients.

OCCUPATION.

A direct connection between this greater susceptibility on the part of the male and the greater average unhealthfulness of his surroundings and habits can be seen in considering the role of occupations as a causative factor.

The avocations of 1,280 patients with laryngeal tuberculosis are shown in the following table:

1. Voice users (actors, singers, elocutionists, hucksters, fakirs, etc.) 71
2. Open air occupations (cabmen, carmen, solicitors, collectors, etc.) 101
3. Laborers and porters......................... 64
4. Clerks, accountants, shop assistants, stenographers, etc. 196
5. Painters 32
6. Students 81
7. Traveling salesmen 40
8. Saloon-keepers, etc. 21
9. Artists (painters, photographers, etc.).......... 14

10. Housewives (laundresses, servants, etc.)......... 203
11. Physicians, dentists and nurses................. 58
12. Dusty occupations (bakers, farriers, stone-cut-
    ters, etc.) 86
13. Sedentary occupations (tailors, shoemakers,
    dressmakers, etc.) 72
14. Machinists, engineers 62
15. Merchants, lawyers, bankers, etc................ 81
16. Farmers 49
17. Musicians—wind instruments 12
19. No occupations 37

                                              1,280

Lake's table, showing the occupations of 200 patients with laryngeal tuberculosis, compared with 200 consecutive cases of phthisis admitted in each of the years 1898 and 1899 to the Mount Vernon Hospital for Consumption, follows:

| | | FIRST 200 CASES | |
| | Laryngeal | — In Years — | |
Occupation	Cases (200)	1898	1899
1. Dusty occupations (bakers, farriers, etc.	50	55	59
2. Sedentary occupations (tailors, shoemakers, etc.	17	21	15
3. Clerks	15	6	9
4. Shop-assistants	12	9	9
5. Waiters	8	5	9
6. Housewives, servants and laundresses	31	43	51
7. Voice users (actors, singers, etc.)	7	2	6
8. Painters	11	12	7
9. Laborers and porters............	26	25	6
10. Open air occupations (cabmen, carmen, etc.)	11	9	18
11. Healthy occupations	12	13	11

While those occupations which are particularly unhealthful show a large percentage of cases with laryngeal involvement, maintaining a relative correspondence to the cases of pulmonary phthisis in the same occupations, it cannot be shown, despite common belief to the contrary, that avocations demanding great vocal strain under unhygienic surroundings, i. e., vaudeville

artists, singers, fakirs, etc., show an unusual percentage, at least in excess of that shown by others living
under the same conditions but not forced to undergo
particular vocal effort. As practically all singers and
fakirs of this class suffer from chronic laryngitis it
would tend to the belief that this condition, so commonly considered a precursor of tuberculosis, can have
but slight determining effect.

Living under the unhygienic conditions of the tenements, etc., does not seem to exert the same deleterious
influence that it does upon lung infection, for throat involvements are found as frequently in people from the
farms and rural communities as from the tenements
and congested areas of the cities.

If tuberculous laryngitis occurred as a primary manifestation of the disease, we would expect to find a
large proportion of the cases from those avocations entailing undue exposure to contagion, independent of the
number of pulmonary cases.

TOBACCO AND ALCOHOL.

Tobacco and alcohol can be at fault in favoring infection only in so far as they are responsible for constitutional and local lessening of tissue resistance. In
moderation they exert no appreciable influence, and
statistics do not show an increased percentage even in
excessive indulgers.

PREVIOUS LOCAL DISEASE.

Some sort of previous disease or abnormal condition
of the laryngeal tissues affected is common, if not invariably essential.

Woodhead, in his lecture before the Henry Phipps Institute in 1905, said:

"The bacillus must make it way not merely onto a free surface, but into the tissues of the body, before it can do any harm; nay, more, it seems that, in the human body at any rate, the tissues must be damaged or weakened and a special mode of entrance into these damaged tissues must be prepared for the tubercle bacillus before it can work its dire effects.

"From my experiments on animals I am satisfied, as are all experimenters, that tuberculosis is never produced without the presence of the tubercle bacillus, but * * * unless the tissues are weakened or damaged, i. e., the soil is prepared, there can be no reaction between the bacillus and the tissues which can end in the production of a tuberculous lesion."

One of the most frequent of these causes of impaired resistance is syphillis. An active lesion is not essential although the secondary infection of such by the tubercle bacillus is frequently observed, but old lesions presumably cured may be as pernicious as the more recent, in that the parts are so weakened as to be susceptible to insults normally impotent.

ACUTE LARYNGITIS.

Acute laryngitis in the phthisical rarely induces the accession of local tuberculosis if the attack be promptly combatted, but neglected attacks or frequent seizures may, under fortuitous conditions, lead to infection or, in healed lesions, to a recurrence.

CHRONIC LARYNGITIS.

In a considerable percentage of cases of laryngeal

phthisis chronic laryngitis exists to a certain degree, independent of, or in connection with pharyngitis and obstructive lesions of the nose. How much influence this chronic inflammation has upon the subsequent development of laryngeal tuberculosis it is impossible to say.

Personally, I have been unable to establish any direct etiologic relationship and, as considered in the discussion of occupations, it is impossible to show that those avocations leading to chronic catarrh show an unduly large proportion of cases of laryngeal phthisis.

NATIONALITY.

All races show an almost equal susceptibility. It has been claimed by some observers, i. e., Norman Bridge (*Tuberculosis*, p. 75, 1903) that: "Nationality has some influence on susceptibility in tuberculosis. The Jewish people have very little of it."

The fallacy of this is readily shown. Of the last 100 cases occurring in the author's practice, 24 were Jews, practically 25 per cent, and these did not include cases resident in the National Jewish Hospital for Consumptives, or the Jewish Consumptives' Relief Society, where there are at all times from fifteen to forty laryngeal cases in a total of some one hundred and fifty patients.

PHYSICAL CHARACTERISTICS.

Certain peculiarities of physique and temperament have been advanced as likely causes of predisposition, but as yet they are little more than theoretical conjectures.

Thost claims to have observed a greater susceptibility on the part of individuals of a tall, slender habit, with long throats and deep voices. I have been unable to find any verification of this.

PREGNANCY.

Child-bearing in consumptives may be the cause of a tuberculous invasion of the larynx through a lighting up of the general process with disseminated infections, or it may lead to the rapid progression of an already existent focus. The strong influence of the parturient state will be seen in the discussion of prognosis.

In conclusion it may be stated as axiomatic that any condition either local or constitutional, leading to impaired vitality of the larynx, renders it more susceptible to invasion by the tubercle bacillus and less resistant to attack when invaded.

CHAPTER V.

PATHOLOGY.

Two groups of phenomena, general and local, follow the advent of tubercle bacilli into the tissues.

The general manifestations, fever, tissue waste, etc., due to the absorption of soluble proteins, belong to the domain of general tuberculosis rather than to a study of the disease as manifest in the larynx.

The local effects are likewise of a dual nature; those consequent upon the action of the bacillus as a simple *corpus alienum,* and those dependent upon its metabolic products and its proteins. As a *corpus alienum,* the bacillus produces changes of a purely inflammatory nature, in large measure of a productive type. The proteins and metabolic products, on the other hand, are responsible for the exudative processes, but in practice it is impossible to differentiate these actions or agencies in considering the tissue changes, for their action is concurrent.

The primary deposit of the bacilli in the larynx, no matter through what channel they may have passed (intact epithelium, erosions, gland ducts, blood or lymphatic vessels) occurs in the sub-epithelial layers of the mucosa and in the sub-mucosa and here their first effects are produced, usually about the blood vessels and glandular acini.

One of four forms of the disease may be provoked: infiltration, ulceration, tuberculoma, or miliary tubercle.

Of these the infiltration and tuberculoma may exist as isolated processes, but the ulcer and miliary tubercle are always preceded and accompanied by other tuberculous conditions.

The Infiltrate:—Pathological and anatomical investigations, as well as clinical observation, establish the fact that every typical tuberculous infection of the larynx begins as an infiltration. Clinically the picture varies with the anatomic peculiarities of the parts involved as well as with the extent of the process, the degree of swelling depending upon the thickness of the submucosa and its relations to the deeper laryngeal structures. In the aryepiglottidean folds, the interarytenoid sulcus and upon the arytenoid cartilages the infiltrate may attain large proportions; on the vocal cords, the lingual surface of the epiglottis and the inner surface of the arytenoids, where there is a scantier supply of submucous tissue, the swelling is usually of moderate extent. The ventricular bands occupy a medium position; the enlargement as a rule is slight, although it may occasionally be sufficient to produce perfect approximation.

Perichondritis is especially liable to occur in those localities where the mucosa is closely adherent to the cartilage, i. e., the epiglottis and arytenoids.

Microscopically an infiltrated area shows the following structure: A normal epithelium, unless the process has advanced to the stage of ulceration or at those points beneath which there is a large aggregation of tubercles, and a subepithelial stratum thickened from two to four times the normal diameter by a deposit of small mononuclear cells, each with a deeply staining nucleus and small protoplasmic body. The primary deposit of these cells usually takes place immediately above the glands, and they are embedded in

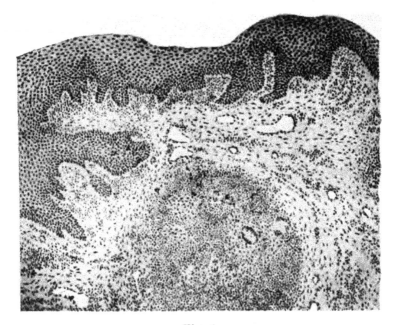

Fig. 1.

a fine or coarse network of connective tissue. Enclosed in this mass there are usually found numerous small and large nodules, or tubercles, the units of which this infiltrated mass is composed. (Fig. 1.)

The Tubercle: As visible macroscopically, the tubercle is a translucent, pearl or grayish colored, spherical body, composed of a cluster of microscopic nodules, the whole forming a body that ranges in size from a mustard seed to a pea. Caseation destroys the translucent appearance and it then becomes opaque and yellow, or a dirty white in color.

The first step in the formation of a tubercle is a proliferation of the endothelial cells of a blood vessel or lymphatic, from which there results a mass of epithelioid cells, so-called because of their resemblance to epithelial cells.

Interspersed among these epithelioid cells are a number of lymphoid cells, separated and enclosed by a sparse fibrillae. The formation within this mass of one or more giant cells completes the typical tubercle,— a rounded nodule, circumscribed and bloodless.

The tubercle formation is most marked in the superficial layers of the mucous membranes, immediately beneath and parallel with the epithelial layer; rarely it extends with even distribution throughout the entire thickness of the mucosa.

In many instances there exists between the epithelial border and the superficial deposit of tubercles a zone of uninvaded tissue, rich in capillaries and containing a few round cells. It was this appearance that led Heinze and Korkunoff to the assumption that the bacilli must be deposited from within by way of the lymphatic and blood vessels.

The Giant Cell:—The giant cell is situated within the tubercle, and is often separated from the small round cells by a collection of large, nucleated, epithelioid cells. These small cells, in gradually decreasing numbers, infiltrate both toward the interior and exterior.

The giant cell itself, a globular body, is composed of

a central mass of granular protoplasm showing some degeneration, and a number of nuclei arranged in a semi-lunar, circular or irregular form around the periphery but probably never in the center. The cell or cells—there may be one or several—occupy either the center or periphery of the tubercle. (Fig. 2.)

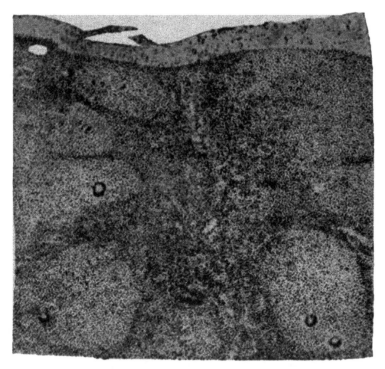

Fig. 2.

The giant cell is frequently found in conditions not tuberculous, i. e., many of the other infectious granulomata, in sarcomata, and in areas chronically irritated by foreign bodies.

In the tubercle they may be very numerous or entirely absent.

The number of tubercles likewise varies, depending

in large measure upon the tissue involved, and hence their absence, together with that of the giant cells, cannot entirely disprove the diagnosis of tuberculosis.

For the same reason the presence of the giant cells alone cannot be taken as an absolute sign of tuberculosis.

Within the tubercle no blood vessels are seen; for a brief period they persist in the tissues between the individual tubercles but even here they soon disappear.

At this stage of development the tubercle commonly undergoes one of two changes—degeneration or organization.

The center of the tubercle begins to show the same condition that has been noted as occurring in the center of the giant cell: the increase in size of the individual tubercle and the conglomeration of the various neighboring tubercles result in shutting off nutrition from the center of the mass, with its consequent destruction, or caseous degeneration.

To this effect the toxic properties of the bacilli contribute. In the course of time this cheesy material liquifies, extends to the surface, breaks through the superficial layers and forms an ulcer. In the lungs this fluid material, after undergoing certain chemical changes, may unite with the lime salts that are dissolved in the blood and are present in the liquid mass, and form calcareous deposits. In the larynx, however, this calcareous degeneration has never been observed. Organization, or fibrous transformation, however, is not rare, and is the method by which the process becomes circumscribed. The areas involved are slowly converted into scar tissue, i. e., fibrous transformation, with encapsulation of the bacilli. If the bacilli are destroyed the disease is cured, otherwise the word arrest is to be employed.

So long as these encapsulated areas, enclosing living bacilli, remain intact, the condition continues quiescent, but subsequent traumatism, through whatever media, may lead to destruction of the protecting wall with breaking down of the old foci or invasion of new areas.

Re-attacks are, therefore, as a rule more severe and harder to combat than the primary.

The Bacilli:—The bacilli in their distribution usually correspond closely to the arrangement of the infiltrated tissues; they are numerous in the deeper layers, more sparsely distributed as the superficial layers are reached and usually entirely absent in the epithelial layer. In the early stage of tubercle evolution the bacilli lie between the epithelioid cells and in the tissues, but later they are situated to a large extent within the cells and especially within the giant cells.

In sections of involved tissue removed endolaryngeally, the bacilli are difficult to demonstrate and rarely more than one or two are to be found even upon prolonged research.

The Ulcer:—The transformation of an infiltrate into an ulcer is due to the caseation of one or more subepithelial tubercles. The tubercles from their primary localization in the submucous tissues extend gradually toward the surface until the epithelial layer is completely detached and destroyed, and the ulcer thus formed enlarges through a continuation of the degenerative process in the individual tubercles, and the coalescense of neighboring ones. (Fig. 3.)

The nature and extent of the individual ulcer depend upon the character and location of the preceeding infiltration. In the beginning it is always superficial unless it has its origin in an infiltrate that involves the glands or glandular layer, in which case it forms a crater-shaped depression with prominent edges, and

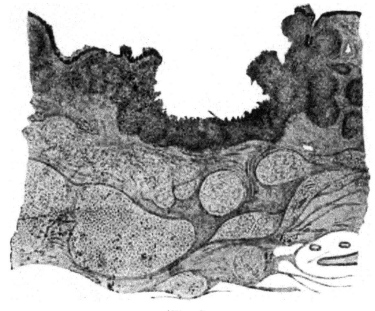

Fig. 3.

may extend to and involve the perichondrium and cartilage.

The variety not situated immediately above the glandular layer is superficial and extends very slowly toward the deeper structures; it has an indefinite border line, irregular, flat or but slightly elevated, and its base is covered by a yellowish exudate through which appear numerous small granulations. If the infiltrate has been extensive the resultant ulcer is generally large and shallow, but if the original deposit was circumscribed and minute, the ulcer is a mere pinhead spot of necrosis.

In all forms of the tuberculous ulcer resulting from infiltration there is present as a typical feature the granulations which cover the base and surround the edges. Occasionally these become exuberant to a degree sufficient to closely resemble papillomata, and almost completely hide the ulcer and fill the glottis.

The "arrosion" or contact ulcers have different characteristics. They are always flat and superficial; they spread rapidly along the surface of the mucosa and have little if any granulation tissue, a marked characteristic of the true ulcer. The exudate which covers the base is thick, tenacious, yellow in color, and sometimes slightly elevated above the level of the surrounding parts.

Tuberculomata:—The tuberculous tumor is one of the rarest manifestations of the disease, but it is impossible to estimate its comparative frequency owing to the fact that there is as yet no strict understanding as to the type of cases to which the term tumor should be applied.

The most satisfactory interpretation of the term is that of Schech (*Handbuch der Laryngologie und Rhinologie*, p. 1144), who understands it to include all tuberculous growths resembling true tumors where the previous existence of an ulcer upon the affected spot can be definitely excluded.

Such growth are most commonly situated upon the posterior wall, in the ventriculus Morgagni and at the anterior commissure. In rarer instances they occur upon the vocal cords the epiglottis and the ventricular bands.

In size they vary from a pin's head to a hickory nut, and may appear singly or in clusters.

Microscopically the tumor is composed of a number of nodules covered by a thickened pavement epithelium.

The individual tubercles consist of numerous small round cells, giant cells and bacilli, and usually show some evidence of caseous degeneration.

The Miliary Tubercle:—The miliary tubercle is rarely seen macroscopically in the larynx, but that the condition does occasionally occur and is clinically recognizable can no longer be denied. Many cases so classed, however, are nothing more than minute granulations, obstructed gland ducts or epithelial abscesses.

The miliary tubercle soon breaks down and ulcerates, but in its early stages it may be seen as an exceedingly minute, gray, yellow or whitish spot gathered in clusters over an infiltrated area or upon the base and around the edges of an ulcer.

The Glands:—Two forms of glandular tuberculosis are recognized: the inter and intra-acinous. In the former there is a multiplication of cells in the connective tissue occupying the spaces between the individual acini, causing their separation and compression, whereby the normal contour is completely destroyed.

The intra-acinous involvement is characterized by a deposit of cells in the acini themselves, ending in complete obliteration.

The Blood Vessels:—Cross section of the blood-vessels shows a pronounced zone of small round cells about the vessels, mostly outside the adventitia but also, to a small extent, invading it, causing an increase of the connective tissue.

Unless the vessel is fully enclosed by a tubercle the muscular layer remains intact even when the adventitia has been destroyed.

Muscles:—Tubercles seldom invade the muscles but that this invasion does exceptionally occur has been demonstrated by Heinze, and Schech has shown their presence in the crico-arytenoideus posticus muscle in a case of tuberculous perichondritis of the cricoid cartilage.

Atrophy of the muscles with fatty and waxy degeneration, due to systemic infection, may occur and produce paralysis.

As will be shown later this condition is sometimes accountable for aphonia in cases of pulmonary phthisis when the larynx is apparently free of disease.

Nerves:—Neuritis and proliferation of the nerve filaments have been described by Dansac (*Annales des Maladies de l'Oreille*, December, 1893). To this condition Gouguenheim gave the name "tubercular pseudoneuroma."

A paralysis is not infrequently seen that may be traced to pressure upon the recurrent laryngeal nerve by enlarged bronchial glands, or in some instances, to the nerve being embedded in an adherent pleura at the apex.

The Mucosa:—Congestion or anemia of the mucous membrane unaccompanied by other evidences of local disease, and frequently classed as tuberculous or pretuberculous catarrh or anemia, cannot with any histologic warrant, be so considered. They are to be classed as "catarrh" or "anemia" accompanying tuberculosis.

With the advance of infiltration the epithelium becomes detached and finally ulcerates, but it remains unaffected in the initial stages, except in the case of arrosion ulcers where superficial necrosis is the primary change.

Chondritis and Perichondritis:—Chondritis, necessarily associated with perichondritis, is a late manifestation developing only when the tuberculous disease has extended to or in the immediate vicinity of the perichondrium.

The cartilages of the larynx are not involved with equal frequency: those most often affected are the arytenoids; then in the order of frequency come the epiglottis, the cricoid and the thyroid. The thyroid, however, according to many observers, is most frequently involved "primarily,"—that is, without demonstrable disease elsewhere.

Mixed Infection:—In the ulcerations other bacteria are usually found, notably the Streptococci and Staphylococci, consequently most ulcers can be considered as depending upon mixed infection. The tubercle bacillus is the first cause, however, and is found in the deeper structures, while the Strepto- and Staphylococci are near or upon the surface.

CHAPTER VI.

SUBJECTIVE SYMPTOMS.

Laryngeal phthisis is accompanied by symptoms so complex that a thoroughly comprehensive view can be obtained only by some such arbitrary classification as the following:

(A.) Subjective symptoms.

(B.) Objective symptoms.

The subjective phenomena are subdivided into two groups:

(C.) Symptoms peculiar to the lungs.

(D.) Symptoms peculiar to the larynx and those common to the lungs and larynx.

The manifestations falling in the latter group (D.) are best considered under two heads:

(1.) Symptoms due to systemic poisoning unassociated with local structural changes of a tuberculous nature.

(2.) Symptoms dependent upon tuberculous cell proliferation in the laryngeal tissues.

(C.) Symptoms peculiar to the lungs:

Except in rare instances the laryngeal symptoms are antedated for variable periods by those dependent upon the lungs, and these do not immediately follow infection;—a sufficient time must elapse in which the bacilli can produce the changes recognized as typical, and this original focus must either produce others or disintegrate with diffusion and absorption of the soluble proteins before constitutional symptoms can appear.

Unfortunately the nature of the process thus precludes the appearance of any distinctive signs until the disease has become fairly well established.

The primary symptoms are usually those of lowered vitality, evidenced by anemia, dyspepsia, loss of weight, appetite, strength, &c. Following—or in some cases primarily—there is cough, with or without expectoration; fever, usually in the afternoon or evening with normal morning remissions; huskiness of the voice or simple voice fatigue; night sweats; hemorrhage; pleuritic pains, &c.

(D.) Symptoms peculiar to the larynx and those common to the lungs and larynx.

(1.) Phenomena not dependent upon structural changes in the larynx:

Certain alterations in the voice, ranging from simple fatigue after prolonged use to complete and lasting aphonia, are occasional symptoms of pulmonary tuberculosis unaccompanied by recognizable laryngeal lesions.

Amblyphonia, or voice weakness, is the most frequent of these phenomena and is usually evidenced by a sense of laryngeal discomfort or fatigue after prolonged reading or speaking. It is an expression of muscular weakness due to anemia or of a lessened expiratory power consequent upon the gradual elimination of certain pulmonary segments.

This last factor naturally becomes more pronqunced in the late stages of the disease. The first and more important factor—muscular weakness—is active in any disease accompanied by rapid or pronounced exhaustion and is therefore not typical of tuberculosis.

Voice fatigue may give way to hoarseness and this in turn be succeeded by aphonia, although there is no regular sequence such as that which usually obtains in true tuberculous laryngitis, for either the aphonia or hoarseness may be primary without any preceding changes. On the other hand the voice may retain its original strength and purity throughout the entire course of the disease, or in case of preceding alterations, may return to its normal state shortly before death.

Either aphonia or amblyphonia may precede all other symptoms of the disease and thus direct attention to the constitutional condition, although they usually develop after the pulmonary process has become well established.

In addition to the etiologic factors already mentioned, muscular weakness and expiratory insufficiency, two other conditions must be taken into consideration: intralaryngeal changes of a non-tuberculous character and tuberculosis of contiguous or extralaryngeal structures.

First among these causes is paralysis of the recurrent laryngeal nerve, which by reason of its long course and varied relationships is especially subject to insult.

In considering the etiology it was shown that involvement of the bronchial glands occurs in nearly all cases of pulmonary phthisis and that in a considerable percentage of all cases they are primarily affected.

Paralysis is frequently due to the pressure of these nodules, or to like action upon the part of the tracheal glands which are situated along the course of the nerve between the trachea and esophagus.

Pleuritic exudates and adhesions may likewise embed the nerves on either side.

Landgraf, Dansac (*Annales des Maladies de l'Oreille*, Dec., 1893) and others have described inflammatory processes in the nerves with proliferation of the nerve filaments which result in paralysis,—the so-called "tubercular pseudo neuroma" of Gouguenheim.

Dansac has found the condition in arytenoid swellings, and Landgraf noted a left recurrent paralysis in which post-mortem examination showed fatty degeneration of both posterior crico-arytenoids, with destruction of the medullary sheath and axis-cylinders of the left nerve.

Although there was a small enlarged gland pressing upon the nerve under the arch of the aorta, he believed the degeneration to be the result of primary inflammation of the neurilemma rather than of pressure.

Atrophy of the laryngeal muscles with fatty or waxy degeneration, either isolated or in common with like changes in the muscles of other organs, has been described by E. Fränkel (*Lehrbuch d. path. gewebelehre,'* 4th edit.) and may be accountable for certain cases of hoarseness. As previously shown, this degeneration is due to the systemic condition and not to local tuberculous infection.

In nearly all cases of pulmonary phthisis there is more or less inflammation of the vocal cords caused by coughing and the constant passage of irritant sputum, with the formation of mucus threads stretching across the glottis from cord to cord, forming a mechanical hindrance to pure tone production and leading to slight, and usually intermittent, attacks of coughing and hoarseness.

A rarer cause is the former occurence of bleeding or pleuritic attacks, leading to voluntary suppression through fear of pain or recurring hemorrhage.

In addition to these manifestations certain other symptoms classed as paresthesias, may develop either concurrent with, or independent of the vocal phenomena.

These sensations, notably those of retained foreign bodies, scratching, tickling and excessive dryness, are referred to either the larynx or pharynx and are practically always provocative of spasmodic attacks of an explosive, or shallow, hacking cough, usually dry but occasionally accompanied by a small amount of frothy mucus. They are an expression of nerve perversion and lowered vitality.

These symptoms, unaccompanied by local tuberculous disease, may disappear spontaneously or by reason of treatment, but usually persist and merge insensibly into the more obstinate symptoms originating in specific cell proliferation. The change is so gradual that it is usually impossible to determine the exact time of transition.

(2.) Symptoms due to specific cell proliferation in the laryngeal tissues:

The advent of a true tuberculous infection is usually soon followed by one or more of a group of symptoms regarded as more or less characteristic, although cases are occasionally seen which progress to death without any momentous subjective manifestations.

The character of the individual symptoms depends more upon the locale of the lesion than upon its type and extent.

For example, in many cases of advanced and widespread extrinsic involvement the purity of tone remains almost unimpaired throughout the entire course of the disease, while on the other hand, moderate infiltration of the interarytenoid sulcus or arytenoid cartilages may lead to complete aphonia. Likewise with dysphagia: a small, shallow ulcer of the epiglottis or aryteno-epiglottidean folds sometimes produces severe and lasting pain, and yet widespread ulceration and infiltration of the vocal cords, interarytenoid sulcus or ventricular bands rarely causes any dysphagia whatsoever. As a general rule it may be said that extrinsic lesions produce pain and that intrinsic involvement causes disturbances of phonation.

VOICE ALTERATIONS:

The hoarseness of tuberculosis is produced by conditions as manifold as the variations in the voice itself.

The typical tuberculous voice is weak, dull, muffled and inflexible, progressing gradually to complete aphonia.

Usually it is less harsh and forcible than the raucous

voice of syphilis, although at times it is impossible to distinguish between the two, for either may depart from the typical and assume the characteristics of the other. It is invariably produced by gross lesions of the cords, infiltrations and ulcerations producing an uneven edge; by inter-arytenoidal swellings, enlarged arytenoids, ankylosis of the crico-arytenoidal joints and extensive infiltrations of the ventricular bands.

Small nodal thickenings on the cords frequently lead to the condition known as diplophonia: a voice generally normal but occasionally broken by sudden changes in pitch. The same condition is met in syphilitic laryngitis and in certain small tumor-like growths, i. e., singers' nodules, polypi, &c.

Moderate infiltration of the cords unaccompanied by ulceration, and lesions leading to imperfect adduction, produce as a rule nothing more serious than slight muffling and premature fatigue.

Large infiltrations of the ventricular bands interfere with tone production to as great an extent as involvement of the true cords.

It is needless to explain why absolutely no inference can be drawn as to the extent or nature of the local lesions from the condition of the voice, although this is a common error of the medical profession as well as of the laity.

In like manner we cannot conclude during the course of treatment, that because of progressive voice destruction, the process is advancing, nor, *per contra*, because of a gradual improvement in phonation that the condition is nearing arrest or undergoing gradual betterment.

Complete cure may result with permanent hoarseness due to a distorted cord, or with a lasting aphonia consequent upon ankylosis or recurrent paralysis; on the other hand, the voice may be regained while lesions of other segments of the larynx, i. e., extrinsic, progress and disintegrate.

Occasionally an atypical case is met, in which there is aphonia with lesions presumably exerting no direct influence upon tone production, and in which the *modus operandi* cannot be satisfactorily explained.

Cough:—Cough practically always accompanies tuberculous laryngeal disease but some few cases escape any except that essential to the removal of sputum. In the early stages it is usually dry, hacking and of a paroxysmal and explosive type; with the advance of the infection it becomes looser and easier though more frequent.

If ulcers are present, particularly of the epiglottis, either isolated or in combination with disease of the aryteno-epiglottidean folds, or if the posterior wall is widely infiltrated, each seizure is attended by severe pain causing efforts at suppression with consequent muffling.

In any given case, no matter what the type of the lesion, it is impossible to form a just estimate as to the exact role played by the larynx for many elements contribute to the production of the phthisical cough.

Naturally it is in large measure due to the lungs—and in so far as the expulsion of secretions is concerned, necessary.

Consideration must likewise be given to such causes as the dropping of saliva or particles of food into the larynx, naso-pharyngeal or pharyngeal catarrh, simple laryngitis and pressure of the vagus.

The "nasal," "stomach," and "nervous" coughs must also be taken into account. The nervous type of cough in particular plays a very important role in these cases.

Granting the importance of these agencies we must still recognize the larynx itself as a not inconsiderable contributory factor.

Certain segments, especially the inter-arytenoid sulcus, are highly sensitive and when diseased respond by outbursts of coughing to the slightest irritation. In phthisis this stimulation is given by previous attacks of coughing and the frequent passage of irritant secretions.

Hypertrophy of the lingual glands, causing contact with the epiglottis, is a not uncommon cause of uncontrollable coughing in many cases. These glands are enlarged to some extent in almost all old cases of pulmonary tuberculosis and in a considerable percentage they are themselves the seat of tuberculous changes.

In this hypersensitive condition of the mucosa many things normally impotent become active irritants, i. e., inhalation of smoke and dust; immoderate use of the voice in speaking, singing or crying; sudden variations in temperature; cold air; strong winds; alcohol; tobacco, &c.

When granulations, irregular growths, rugous infiltrations or ulcers exist, the secretions cling tenaciously to their uneven surfaces and lead frequently to prolonged attacks of coughing, so severe as to leave the patient completely exhausted and fighting for breath.

SECRETIONS.

In the late stages of the disease the lungs pour into the already diseased larynx such colossal quantities of irritant secretions that the cough becomes almost incessant and adds much to the already intolerable conditions. The inflamed laryngeal mucosa itself excretes considerable mucus, but not sufficient to occasion any particular distress in its expulsion unless there is simultaneous discharge from the lungs.

With widespread ulceration there is produced a thin, dirty white, and occasionally bloody pus, mixed with mucus and dead epithelial cells, which has a peculiarly sour, penetrative odor.

In cases of perichondrial abscesses the breath is foul and small fragments of cartilage may be found in the secretions.

Small hemorrhages from ulcerated areas or exuberant granulations are sometimes noted but true bleeding almost never occurs from the larynx. I have seen but one such case, a young man with deep ulceration of the right ventricular band from which bleeding occurred on two separate occasions, the quantity each time amounting to between two and three drams. After thorough cleansing the blood could be seen exuding from the ulcerated area.

FEVER.

Laryngeal tuberculosis may cause considerable fever at times, as is shown by an increase of the daily range coincident with the breaking down of new areas or extension of old lesions.

A temperature of 100 to 101 degrees occasionally ac-

companies acute cases where the pulmonary process
has been for some time quiescent, but as a rule, unless
the local process is associated with considerable acute
inflammation, a comparatively rare condition, the temperature is not much affected by the laryngeal invasion. After endolaryngeal operations the temperature rises from one to three degrees, then gradually re-
cedes until it is again normal by the end of two or
three, or occasionally four days.

DYSPHAGIA.

True dysphagia occurs, as a rule, only when the
laryngeal condition is well advanced.

In 904 personally observed cases of laryngeal phthisis, dysphagia occurred at some period of the disease
in 247, or 27.32 per cent.

The term dysphagia, as here used, includes all varieties—odynophagia or painful deglutition; dysphagia
or obstructed swallowing, and the entrance of food and
liquids into the larynx.

The conditions practically always coexist and in
large measure depend upon like pathologic conditions,
hence the propriety of considering them under the common appellation of dysphagia.

The appearance of this symptom must always be
considered ominous, both because it marks an extension
of the process with probable involvement of the deeper,
or more vulnerable structures, and because, unless
promptly controlled, the consequent enforced reduction
or withdrawal of food leads to rapid collapse.

Dysphagia is an invariable consequence of all widespread involvements of the upper aperture of the

larynx, i. e., epiglottis and aryteno-epiglottidean folds.

Moderate infiltrations, or small-sized ulcerations of the epiglottis and aryteno-epiglottidean folds may be unaccompanied by pain, but when either process is moderately advanced each act of swallowing is accomplished at the expense of such excruciating and unbearable suffering that starvation seems the lesser evil.

Extensive infiltrations of the posterior wall or arytenoid cartilages, and perichondritis or perichondrial abscesses, are almost as potent in the production of pain. In all such cases the passage of liquids is usually more difficult than the swallowing of solid and semiliquid food.

Involvements of the middle larynx, whether ulcerative or infiltrative, cause pain only in exceptional cases. Chordal lesions do not produce dysphagia and the ventricular bands are responsible only when the lesion is acute or widespread. Acute, lancinating pain nearly always characterizes the outbreak of miliary tubercles.

In addition to the painful and difficult deglutition, there is frequently added a sharp, neuralgic-like pain in the ear of the corresponding side or in both ears in bilateral lesions, by transference through the auricular branch of the vagus. This aural pain occurs, at some period, in practically all dysphagic cases.

In rarer instances the pain is referred to the salpingo-pharyngeal fold and palate.

Rigidity of the muscles, particularly of the posterior wall and epiglottis, leading to imperfect closure during deglutition, permits both solids and liquids to enter the larynx with violent cough and laryngeal spasm.

Actual destruction of tissue plays no role in this for

deglutition can occur normally after complete removal or destruction of the epiglottis.

The pain depends upon various causes:—when ulcers exist it is due to the mechanical, thermic and chemical action of the passing food and secretions upon the exposed nerve endings, but in the absence of ulceration it may be ascribed to rigidity, to pressure of the inflamed tissues and muscles, to neuritis and to perichondritis.

Pain may likewise be caused by speaking or coughing through the movement produced in the affected tissues. Many patients also complain of a constant ache or soreness in the throat independent of any muscular action.

Intimately associated with the various types of dysphagia is a symptom almost totally overlooked in works on laryngeal phthisis, yet it is one that is responsible for extreme discomfort and annoyance: the regurgitation of fluid and solid food through the nose.

In 247 cases of dysphagia, regurgitation occurred at some period of the disease in 198, over 80 per cent.

Even when the pain is not severe, this factor if pronounced may necessitate, for the time being, the almost complete withdrawal of food.

DYSPNEA.

Shortness of breath is the rule in advanced cases of phthisis, but true dyspnea of a degree sufficient to occasion alarm, dependent upon intralaryngeal swelling, is the most uncommon of the special symptoms, and usually occurs only in those cases where treatment has been neglected or where an acute inflammation has been superadded to the chronic process.

In any case sudden dyspnea may result, due to edema, abscess formation, perichondritis or paralysis of the abductors.

The last cause is well exemplified by the following case:

Miss S., *act* 29, nurse, was first seen in April, 1904, when the larynx presented the following picture: both cords extensively ulcerated and infiltrated; ventricular bands partially overlap the cords and are deeply ulcerated; right arytenoid edematous with a small ulcer on its inner surface.

During the following nine months the condition rapidly improved and by January, 1905, there remained only moderate infiltration of the cords with fixation of the right cord in the median line. At this time she had an attack of pleurisy with a large effusion on the left side and it was not until several weeks later that she again appeared for examination.

The larynx was unaltered and the breathing fairly easy, considering the medium fixation of the right cord and the labored heart action due to the large pleural effusion.

The following day, while resting quietly, she was attacked by sudden dyspnea and examination revealed total bilateral abductor paralysis. Tracheotomy was immediately performed but death ensued eleven hours later. No autopsy was held.

Dyspnea of slow development, the essentially chronic type, may depend upon any one or more of a variety of conditions; a distorted or greatly infiltrated epiglottis; swelling of the aryteno-epiglottidean folds with simultaneous enlargement of the arytenoid cartilages; bilateral infiltration of the ventricular bands; ankylosis of the cricoarytenoids; abductor paralysis; subchordal swellings; excessive granulations and tuberculomata.

The formation of cicatricial bands between the cords is a rare factor and in all likelihood depends upon the existence of a mixed lesion, syphilis and tuberculosis, for the latter disease alone rarely leads to the formation of scar tissue to any considerable extent.

Ordinarily the process does not advance to the point of complete closure; by the time the breathing has become labored the general disease has advanced so far that the patient succumbs, if not, endolaryngeal surgical and medicinal treatment will usually cause some retrogression.

The cases in which tracheotomy is necessitated are exceedingly rare, and will become ever rarer as the infections are more universally recognized in the early stages and therefore are more rationally and persistently treated.

CHAPTER VII.

OBJECTIVE SYMPTOMS.

Infiltration is the first objective sign of laryngeal phthisis. Nearly all observers speak of a tuberculous or pre-tuberculous catarrh as the first and therefore the mildest form of laryngitis, but the assumption of such a condition is entirely without warrant.

CATARRH.

Many cases of pulmonary phthisis show a more or less catarrhal condition of the laryngeal mucosa. This chronic congestion depends upon one or more of several factors; lowered vitality; cough; passage of sputum; disturbed digestion; naso-pharyngeal catarrh, etc.. Neither must it be forgotten that the unhygienic conditions which predispose the individual to pulmonary tuberculosis likewise predispose to chronic catarrhal laryngitis.

While the frequency of this early catarrh must be admitted, there is in fact no reason for assuming it to be tuberculous and even less for considering it "pre-tuberculous." Unless it can be shown that it later evolves into true tuberculosis the use of this latter term cannot be defended, and this transformation, it can be most emphatically stated, does not occur.

Bacillary infection may take place in catarrhal

membranes the same as in normal membranes, but a conversion of a simple catarrh into tuberculosis never occurs.

Many of the cases of so-called tuberculous catarrh are in reality incipient tuberculous infiltrates, as can be demonstrated by the injection of tuberculin, which produces a visible increase of hyperemia and swelling with the occasional eruption of miliary tubercles.

The clinical history in such a case is different from that of a simple inflammation; the congested areas are more resistant to treatment, commonly affect only one side of the larynx and if neglected advance to localized tumefaction and possibly ulceration.

The most common site of the early infiltrate is the interarytenoid sulcus and here the differential diagnosis between early tuberculous infiltration and simple catarrhal thickening is exceedingly difficult, for it is also one of the points of election for the latter condition.

The most characteristic feature of the tuberculous hyperemia is its tendency to affect only one-half of the larynx while the catarrhal congestion is always bilateral.

Redness of one cord, arytenoid, ventricular band, etc., is generally indicative of one of four conditions: tuberculosis, syphilis, malignancy or traumatism, and the differential diagnosis depends upon the accompanying conditions and personal history.

ANEMIA.

Perhaps the most widespread of all the fallacies concerning laryngeal phthisis is that respecting the diagnostic significance of palatal, pharyngeal and laryngeal pallor.

The commonly accepted view is thus expressed by J. Solis Cohen:

"Congestion of the mucous membrane almost always marks the earliest recognizable stage of the acuter form, while pallor of the mucous membrane almost always characterizes the earliest recognizable stage of the chronic and more frequent form."

This early laryngeal pallor, it is claimed, is independent of general pallor and is frequently associated with anemia of the pharynx, palate and mouth.

While the diagnostic worth of this sign has been almost universally acclaimed, it merits, according to the author's experience, but slight consideration. Its frequency in the early stages of the chronic variety of phthisis has been greatly exaggerated as is shown by the following table based upon six hundred cases of comparatively early lesions:

Total number of cases, 600.

	Normal.	Anemic.	Hyper-emic.	
Palatal Mucosa	264	129	207	600
Laryngeal Mucosa	38	95	467	600
Total	302	224	674	1200

In this table, in so far as possible, every unusually acute case has been eliminated.

These statistics show that pallor of the mucosa is far less frequent than congestion even in the essentially chronic cases. The proportion is about 1 to 3. In the far advanced cases the percentage showing anemia is necessarily much larger.

Moreover, in nearly all cases in which this anemia

was present, its value in diagnosis was almost *nil*, as other signs existed which made clear the condition without considering the pallor, and in the majority of instances the pallor was not localized in the larynx or mouth but was simply an expression of general anemia, the conjunctiva, etc., showing like changes.

Even the first stage of pulmonary tuberculosis, the so-called "apical catarrh," is almost always associated with signs of general anemia. In these cases, according to Grawitz and Strauer, the red cells are reduced and the clinical picture is that of pseudo-chlorosis.

A like condition of the laryngeal mucosa is found in many normal individuals in whom tuberculosis does not later develop; it is almost invariably present in general anemia and may be general or of localized areas. It is an expression of the various wasting diseases, diarrhea, etc., and a grayish white color of the interarytenoidal mucosa is found in many cases of simple chronic catarrh, due to necrosis of the epithelial layer.

Certain tuberculous lesions of an advanced type, flabby granulations, warty growths, old infiltrations and edematous swellings may be pale and anemic, but the areas surrounding and separating the individual lesions are usually somewhat congested.

It may be said then, that the pallor of laryngeal phthisis is nothing more than an expression of general tissue waste, and that as such it should lead to further investigation as to its probable origin,—but that it is not pathognomonic of phthisis, is not distnctive and not even suggestive, except as any expression of general anemia may be so considered.

Both the initial catarrh and anemia, unless the former can be shown to depend on infiltration, should be classed as catarrh or anemia accompanying tuberculosis and not as a tuberculous or pre-tuberculous catarrh or anemia.

Excluding these two conditions four forms of laryngeal phthisis are clinically demonstrable.

1. The infiltrate.
2. The ulcer.
3. The tumor.
4. The miliary tubercle.

Certain subdivisions have been attempted, such as the "*scléreuse et végétante*" of Gouguenheim and Glower, the "*forme dysphagique*" of Ferrand and Bovet, the hypertrophic form, etc., but such a multiplication of terms is inadvisable as they are not distinctive types but merely variations of the primary groups. Granulations, likewise, are a result of ulceration and are not to be looked upon as a distinct variety.

Except in rare instances the individual case does not conform exactly to any one of the four types; two or more coexist.

In the incipient stages infiltration alone is generally present but with advance of the process some point gives way and ulceration complicates the picture.

The true tumor, alone of the other forms, exists as an uncomplicated entity. The miliary type is generally found in connection with ulceration and infiltration.

1. The INFILTRATION.

Infiltration is the earliest and most characteristic of the objective symptoms, and may persist indefinitely without degeneration or the development of other signs of local infection.

Commonly, after a shorter or longer interval, the superficial layers of the mucosa succumb to the con-

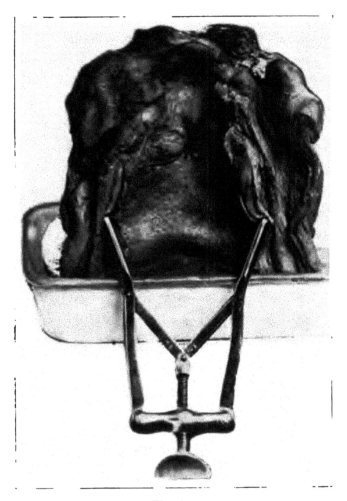

Fig. 4.

stantly increasing pressure of the subepithelial exudate and to the gradual obliteration of the blood vessels, and the characteristic ulcer appears.

In the beginning the infiltrate, especially if it is limited to the posterior ends of the true cords or to the interarytenoid sulcus, may strongly resemble simple catarrhal laryngitis, but in the majority of the cases, however, we do not have to deal with such an isolated simple process for there is usually an early extension to neighboring structures and contiguous tissues, until finally the entire larynx, or a large portion thereof, is involved, either with or without concomitant ulceration. (Fig. 4.)

Interarytenoid Sulcus: Infiltration of the inter-arytenoidal mucosa is the most frequent and pathognomonic localization of the earlier manifestations of the disease, and often persists unaltered and uncomplicated for many months or years. The comparative frequency of this type is shown in the following table:

Author.	Cases.	Inter-arytenoid Infiltration.	Isolated Interarytenoid Lesions.
Keller	48	34	8
Carmody	81	71	7
Author	904	640	79
Total	1033	745	94

In the early stages of the disease the sulcus is partially filled by a circumscribed swelling which forms a convex projection during deep inspiration. The growth may occupy any part of the incisure; it is usually in the middle, more seldom upon one side infringing upon the corresponding cord, and occasionally upon each side giving to the middle portion a sunken, punched out appearance.

The size and character of the infiltrate also varies within wide extremes; in the simplest type it forms a broad-based, more or less elevated, red or grayish white projection covered by a smooth or slightly uneven epithelium. (Plate I, Fig. 5.)

The grayish white color depends upon necrosis of the superficial epithelium and is not distinctive of tuberculosis for it also obtains in other conditions.

The pallor, therefore, cannot be considered as diagnostic unless it covers a convex infiltrate—and then it is the peculiar character of the swelling and not the pallor that is distinctive. In some cases the growth is an angry red in color.

The infiltrate frequently departs from this early type and takes on the characteristics of a tumor; it is sharply circumscribed, with wide base and pointed extremity, and projects slightly into or almost completely fills the space between the vocal cords. (Plate I, Fig. 6.)

The free edge of this tumor-like body may be comparatively smooth or distinctly rugous, i. e., covered by numerous sharp, ragged, tooth-like projections.

In rare instances the infiltrate may somewhat resemble papillomata, the so-called "vegetierende" or "papillaere" forms. (Plate I, Fig. 7.)

Vocal Cords: Infiltration of the vocal cords, in the early stages, is marked by a diffuse or circumscribed redness and moderate swelling strongly suggestive of simple chronic laryngitis.

The tuberculous hyperemia, however, has a decided tendency to involve only one cord or isolated portions thereof, or if bilateral, both sides are rarely involved to an equal extent, in contrast with the symmetrical

PLATE I.

FIG. 5.   Broad-based infiltrate of the posterior wall.

FIG. 6.   Tumor-like infiltrate of the posterior wall.

FIG. 7.   Papillomatous infiltrate of the posterior wall.

PLATE I.

Fɪɢ. 5. Tuberculous infiltrate of the posterior wall.

Fɪɢ. 6. Tumor-like infiltrate of the posterior wall.

Fɪɢ. 7. Papillomatous-like infiltrate of the posterior wall.

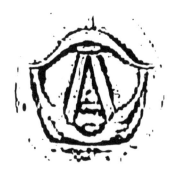

Fig. 5.

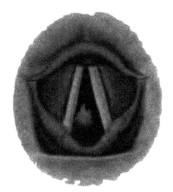

Fig. 6.

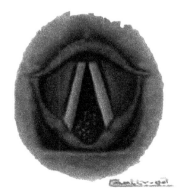

Fig. 7.

PL

and bilateral distribution of the non-specific inflammations.

The circumscribed infiltrations are most common on the vocal processes, and are generally found in connection with hyperplasia of the interarytenoidal mucosa. In such cases the posterior ends of the cords are of a pink or deep red color, somewhat uneven or notched along the free edge and rounded in form with an apparent increase both in width and thickness.

If the ligamentous portion remains free the condition has some resemblance to pachydermia and a microscopic examination, if other symptoms are lacking, may be the only means of determining the nature of the process.

Before the infiltrate has attained sufficient volume to produce evident increase in size the only alteration is in color, either as a redness or a loss of the normal pearly lustre. Even this slight change, particularly when limited to one cord, is highly suggestive.

In rare instances the anterior commissure is the site of a circumscribed infiltrate which affects either the angle of the cords or the region immediately above or below it. Even when moderate such a thickening interferes with perfect adduction and vocalization.

The circumscribed infiltrations rarely persist for any considerable time without involving the mid-section of the cord and when this occurs the appearance is almost pathognomonic; the cord becomes cylindrical in form, convex from free edge to inner margin and from end to end, whereby the mid-section appears considerably wider than the extremities. (Plate 2, Fig. 8.)

The surface may show a number of oblique dilated vessels and the color is either a dull or beefy red. The cord is sometimes thickened to many times its normal diameter, completely closing the ventricle and obliterating the line between the cord and ventricular band; in such cases the border between the two is indicated by a thin dark line.

Frequently the free edge of the cord is furrowed by a longitudinal groove through the pressure exerted by the opposite cord.

The same condition is simulated by marked swelling of both the inferior and superior surface of the cords, due to the close connection between the free edge and the muscular layer whereby it is prevented from swelling to a degree equal to that of the other segments.

Arytenoid Cartilages: Isolated infiltration of the arytenoid cartilages is comparatively common, but frequently there is simultaneous involvement of the ary-epiglottic folds.

In the early stages the process is mostly unilateral, in the advanced bilateral, and shows as a single or double pear-shaped mass of deep red or purplish color, the extremities of which extend upward and outward until lost in the ary-epiglottic fold. (Plate 2, Fig. 9.)

If the infiltrate is of long standing and large proportions the mucosa becomes pale and translucent, the interarytenoid sulcus partially obliterated and Wrisberg's cartilage hidden. Movement of the cords is mechanically hindered by the enlarged cartilage as well as by ankylosis of the crico-arytenoidal joint. Acute inflammatory swelling of one or both arytenoids

PLATE II.

FIG. 8. Infiltration of the vocal cords and interarytenoid sulcus. The cords have assumed the typical cylindrical form.

FIG. 9. Infiltration and congestion of the right arytenoid cartilage and ventricular band. The corresponding cord is ulcerated along the free edge and somewhat thickened.

FIG. 10. Edema and colossal swelling of both arytenoid cartilages.

PLATE II.

FIG. 8. Cylindrical vocal cords.

FIG. 9. Ulceration of the right vocal cord and infiltration of the corresponding arytenoid and ventricular band.

FIG. 10. Edema of the arytenoid cartilages.

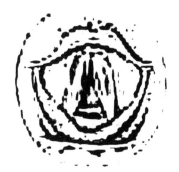

Fig. 8.

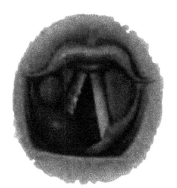

Fig. 9.

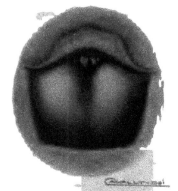

Fig. 10.

PLATE II.

during the course of chronic tuberculous inflammation frequently occurs.

Aryteno-epiglottidean Folds: In these folds in-filtration reaches a high degree owing to the abundant loose, submucous tissue. It is usually bilateral but may be limited to one side, and is always found in combination with either arytenoidal or epiglottic disease, and frequently both.

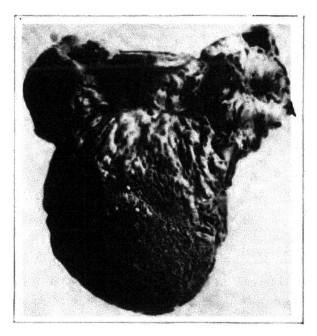

Fig. 11.

In connection with bilateral arytenoidal swelling the appearance is absolutely pathognomonic. On either side the pyriform or flask-shaped tumors encroach upon the lumen of the upper aperture, which is still further closed by the enormous globular masses representing the arytenoids proper which meet in the middle line posteriorally and extend back into the pharynx.

There is usually some edema present giving to the otherwise red body a pale and translucent appearance. Such cases generally have a fatal termination and their course is attended by severe dysphagia and some dyspnea. (Plate 2, Fig. 10.)

Epiglottis: Widespread infiltration of the epiglottis, in the great majority of instances, is a late manifestation although now and then it is met as an early or even the primary laryngeal focus.

In the milder forms the edge is swollen to several times the normal thickness and has the appearance of being rolled upon itself; the color may be either bright red or pale. (Fig. 11.)

The swelling is often almost as great as that of the ary-epiglottic folds, giving it the so-called "turban" or "omega" shape. (Plate III, Fig 12.)

The infiltration is sometimes limited to one half the organ (Plate III, Fig. 13.) and I have had occasion to observe several unusual cases in which there has been no swelling except in the space between the epiglottis and base of the tongue, extending, with gradually decreasing distinctness, toward the free edge.

Severe pain almost always marks epiglottic involvement and even slight infiltration destroys its mobility.

Ventricular Bands: A considerable percentage of all cases of tuberculous laryngitis show some infiltration of the ventricular bands, which may be the first localization of the process in the larynx. As a rule it is of moderate extent but occasionally reaches large proportions.

In the latter case the vocal cord of the corresponding

PLATE III.

FIG. 12. "Turban" or "Omega" shaped epiglottis. Both cords show slight ulceration and the arytenoid cartilages are uneven and nodular. .

FIG. 13. Warty infiltration of the left side of the epiglottis. The corresponding arytenoid is slightly thickened, the interarytenoid sulcus infiltrated, and both cords congested.

FIG. 14. Bilateral infiltration of the ventricular bands. The left vocal cord and interarytenoidal mucosa are slightly ulcerated.

PLATE III.

Fig. 12.   Turban-shaped epiglottis.

Fig. 13.   Warty infiltration of the epiglottis.

Fig. 14.   Bilateral infiltration of the ventricular bands.

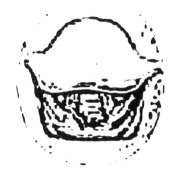

Fig. 12.

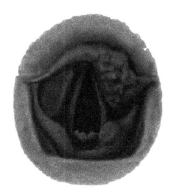

Fig. 13.

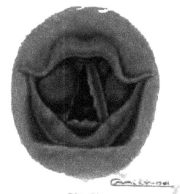

Fig. 14.

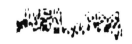

side may be completely hidden; if of less extent one or both ends of the cords remain visible. (Plate III, Fig. 14.)

In bilateral swelling the bands sometimes meet in the median line, causing some dyspnea and aphonia, or usurping the functions of the true cords when these are destroyed, they produce a rough, suppressed voice. The anterior wall of the larynx is involved in a small proportion of the cases.

Subglottic Region: With the exception of the form known as "chorditis vocalis inferior" or "laryngitis hypoglottica," infiltrations in the subglottic region are rare.

Laryngitis hypoglottica conveys the impression of an extra vocal cord parallel with and slightly beneath the true cord. It is either single or bilateral, and of a bright or pale red color, and originates either from an extension of the infiltrate from the inferior surface of the true cords or by primary deposit.

Instead of forming distinct bands the infiltrate may almost completely encircle the larynx. (Plate IV, Fig. 15.)

2. THE ULCER.

As infiltration is considered the first objective sign of laryngeal phthisis, so ulceration may be looked upon as the second distinctive manifestation.

Other conditions sometimes intervene between the ·stages of infiltration and ulceration, or the latter may never occur, but in the average progressive case such a sequence is the rule.

The typical ulcer is always dependent upon infiltration through the disintegration of caseated tubercles, and the first changes occur in the subepithelial tissues.

There is another variety, however, of characteristic appearance, due to sputal infection, that of necessity begins in the epithelium itself. The first of these is marked by three characteristics: the ill-defined margins, irregular and uneven, the so-called worm-eaten appearance; the presence of granulations and of miliary tubercles.

The edges are occasionally prominent and partially overlap and obscure the base, hence the true size and limits of the ulcer cannot always be definitely determined.

The second and more pathognomonic peculiarity is the presence of numerous small, red granulations upon the floor and around the margins of the ulcers.

The third, and absolutely diagnostic feature, is the small grayish or yellowish spot known as the miliary tubercle.

The base is almost always covered by a tenacious yellowish or dirty white exudate of pus and dead epithelial cells.

The most frequent sites of such ulcers are the vocal cords, interarytenoid sulcus, arytenoid cartilages and epiglottis. They occur as well, however, upon all segments of the larynx.

The type of the resultant ulcer depends in large measure upon the locality involved; in segments rich in glands and covered by cylindrical epithelium it is deeper and more crater-like in form than where it involves areas covered by pavement epithelium. Ex-

PLATE IV.

PLATE IV.

Fig. 15. Subglottic infiltration.

Fig. 16. Ulcerated infiltrate of the interarytenoid sulcus.

Fig. 17. Ulceration at corresponding points of both cords.

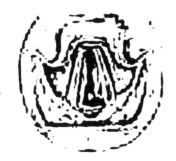

Fig. 15.

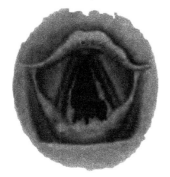

Fig. 16.

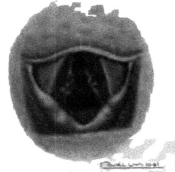

Fig. 17.

PLATE IV.

PLATE IV.

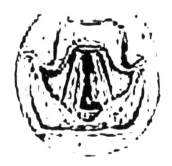

Fig. 15.

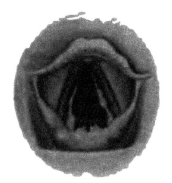

Fig. 16.

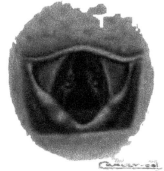

Fig. 17.

PLATE IV.

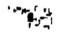

tension occurs through confluence of contiguous ulcers and the slow superficial extension of the individual areas.

Arrosion Ulcers: Non-tuberculous ulcers may occur in the larynges of phthisical subjects the same as in other inflammatory conditions and heal without subsequent infection by the bacillus, as is shown by their occasional prompt disappearance under simple treatment, but early invasion of the necrotic areas by the tubercle bacilli, however, is so constant that it is a safe rule to regard all such ulcers as tuberculous.

The superficial tuberculous ulcers, due primarily to the action of the irritant sputum with early bacillary infection, occur mostly upon the tip of the epiglottis, the vocal cords, inner sides of the arytenoids and the posterior and lateral walls of the trachea, and are usually found in connection with widespread pulmonary involvement with profuse secretions.

They appear at numerous points or in groups of two or more, are essentially superficial and are round, oblong or irregular in shape, the edges are sharp and brilliantly inflamed, and they spread with great rapidity, largely through the confluence of contiguous foci. The base is covered by an elevated membrane strongly resembling that due to diphtheria, and the granulations of the true ulcer are lacking.

While the clinical picture is usually distinctive, it is not possible, without histologic demonstration of miliary tubercles about or on the base, to definitely determine their true nature.

That ulcers of this type exist in the larynges of tuberculous individuals is strongly denied by many

modern observers, but what other theory will explain
their rapid cicatrization which occurs frequently after
simple treatment and oftimes even spontaneously?

Moreover, as has already been shown, ulcers of a
like nature are sometimes found in the air passages
of individuals to whom no suspicion of phthisis can
attach, and upon other mucous membranes as well. and
why, therefore, should the possibility of their occurrence in the larynges of consumptives, where all the
conditions favorable to their development are present,
be denied?

The character of the individual ulcer, whatever the
type, depends upon the nature of the tissue involved
and, therefore, can be best described by taking up in
turn the various segments of the larynx as was done
in the discussion of infiltrations.

Interarytenoid Sulcus: As the posterior wall
is one of the points of election for infiltration so it
is likewise a favored site for ulceration. The early
ulcer is frequently overlooked because the prominent
borders or large granulations about the edges partially
obscure it unless the methods of Killian or Kirstein
are used. For the same reason the necrosis is generally much more extensive than is apparent in the
reflected image.

The first visible change in the infiltrated tissue is a
gradual grayish or bluish white discoloration of the
convex border, due to the pressure of the subepithelial
exudate with resultant necrosis on the surface.

As this gives way the formerly more or less smooth
surface becomes indented by deep clefts, giving rise
to the so-called "saw tooth" appearance, or if only

PLATE V.

FIG. 18. Ulceration of the free edges of the vocal cords, giving the so-called "saw-tooth" appearance.

FIG. 19. Cleft cord.

FIG. 20. Chorditis granulosa.

PLATE V.

Fig. 18. "Saw tooth" cords.

Fig. 19. Cleft cord.

Fig. 20. Chorditis granulosa.

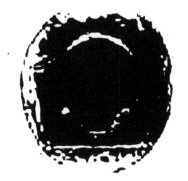

Fig. 18.

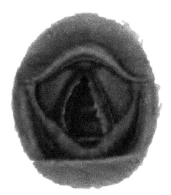

Fig. 19.

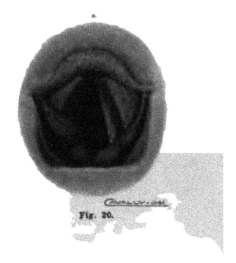

Fig. 20.

PLATE V.

the middle surface is involved, the convex edge appears as though a portion had been removed by a punch.

The base shows numerous small red granulations that about the edges reach a considerable size and extend like sharp ragged teeth into the lumen of the larynx. (Plate IV, Fig. 16.)

These granulations ulcerate in turn and are surrounded by new granulations, giving the impression of "a chain of mountains with narrow valleys running between them."—Friedrich.

In cases running a rapid course the granulations may be so extensive and numerous as to strongly resemble papillomata, or in other instances they become edematous and almost fill the glottis.

Vocal Cords: Ulceration of the interarytenoidal mucosa is nearly always complicated by some destruction of the vocal cords and particularly of their posterior ends.

Frequently this cord necrosis is hidden by overlapping granulations of the posterior wall and come into view only when these are removed; in other instances the yellowish exudate covering most of the necrotic areas, if the ulcer is shallow, gives the impression of a normal condition.

The ulcers vary in characteristics according to their location upon the cord, the free edge, upper or inferior surface.

In many cases they occur upon symmetrical points of both cords, generally at the point of juncture of the middle and anterior third. (Plate IV, Fig. 17.)

On the free edge there may be one or more small necrotic points separated by areas of apparently normal or infiltrated tissue, or the entire margin may be converted into a long, narrow, irregular slough completely destroying the normal contour of the cord. (Plate V, Fig. 18.)

Upon the vocal processes there is a characteristic type in which upon the most prominent point of the infiltrate a hollowing or reaming-out occurs, forming a triangular defect with the apex anterior. The edges are smooth and clear-cut and the base yellow in color. It is this form which bears such a marked resemblance to pachydermia but in the latter disease true ulceration never occurs.

An ulcer occasionally forms in the groove formed along the edge of the infiltrated cord by the pressure of the opposite band, and gives to it a cleft or divided appearance. (Plate V, Fig. 19.)

Schech has described a case of complete separation of the cord from the vocal process.

Because of the small amount of submucous tissue at this point and the superficial position of the arytenoid cartilage, ulcers of the vocal processes frequently lead to perichondritis.

Ulcers occasionally form along the entire upper surface of the cord converting it into a series of longitudinal folds; if the free edge and inner margin are involved the uninvaded middle portion projects prominently above the level of the remaining segments; if the middle section only is ulcerated the margins appear somewhat elevated.

Besides these definite types there are many others of various forms—mostly round, oval or irregular.

Ulcerations on the inferior surfaces of the cords

are not uncommon, but are rarely recognized until they have reached large proportions or until the accompanying granulations extend beyond the free edges. The granulations occasionally become so ex-

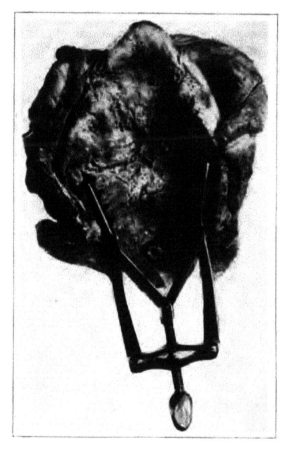

Fig. 21.

cessive as to completely cover the cord or to fill the glottis sufficiently to produce dyspnea.

In certain cases the upper surface is studded with small granulations leading to the condition known as "chorditis granulosa." They occasionally resemble a string of beads strung along the inner margin of the cord. (Plate V, Fig. 20.)

Epiglottis: Infiltration of the epiglottis is almost always soon followed by ulceration. (Fig. 21). The laryngeal surface is the favored site but the free edge is also frequently attacked, especially by that type known as the aphthous or arrosion ulcer. If such occur the entire free edge is dotted with small, flat, white, smooth points of necrosis.

The intermediate mucosa is red and swollen and the whole surface is bathed in tenacious muco-pus.

The deeper ulcers lead to marked distortion and destruction of the entire organ.

Contrary to the commonly accepted view that tuberculosis rarely leads to complete destruction, in contrast with syphilis (*Schech, Lake and others*), it has been the author's experience that the entire organ may melt away with great rapidity. At the present time he has under occasional observation a man of 29 years in whom there is only a small stump representing what formerly was the epiglottis. The organ was entirely destroyed in the winters of 1903 and 1904 and complete arrest ensued. A considerable number of such cases have been seen. (Plate VI, Fig. 22.)

Instances in which the entire free edge or one-half of the organ has disappeared are relatively common in advanced cases. (Plate VI, Fig. 23.)

Defects, such as "V" shaped incisures, etc., are often seen. (Plate VI, Fig. 24.)

If limited to the lower part of the laryngeal surface the ulcers may at times be recognized with difficulty owing to the immobility consequent upon widespread

PLATE VI.

FIG. 22. Almost complete destruction of the epiglottis The process was arrested and did not recur despite subsequent infection of the arytenoids, the aryepiglottic folds and the ventricular bands.

FIG. 23. Destruction of the entire right half of the epiglottis.

FIG. 24. "V" shaped defect in the epiglottis due to circumscribed ulceration, with extensive ulceration of the corresponding arytenoid.

PLATE VI.

FIG. 22.   Complete destruction of the epiglottis.

FIG. 23.   Destruction of one-half the epiglottis.

FIG. 24.   "V" shaped defect of the epiglottis.

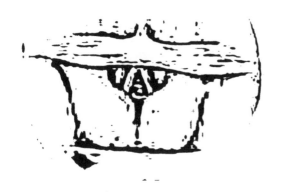

Fig. 22.

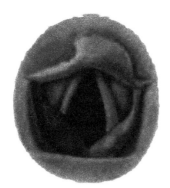

Fig. 23.

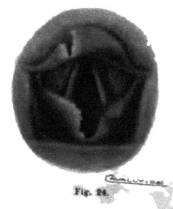

Fig. 24.

PLATE VI.

infiltration, to the overhang of a rounded edge or to exuberant granulations. These obstacles can usually be overcome; if not, the epiglottis can be retracted, or a pledget of cotton swept over the hidden surface may show blood.

Primary ulceration of the lingual surface is one of the rarest manifestations of the disease and I have seen but one such case, combined in this instance with ulceration of the base of the tongue. (Plate VII, Fig. 25.) In several additional cases there was ulceration of the lingual surface secondary to extensive disease of the laryngeal surface and free edge.

Widespread epiglottic involvement is usually secondary to other laryngeal foci but occurs occasionally as the primary localization.

An hitherto unobserved type of laryngeal involvement was recently brought to the author's attention by Dr. T. E. Carmody. The lingual glands were somewhat swollen, there was moderate infiltration of the Lig. Glosso-Epiglotticum, and the free edge of the epiglottis was greatly thickened and rolled upon itself, making a sigmoid curve.

The unique feature consisted of two complete perforations, the one located at the tongue border a little to the right of the median line, the other near the middle and somewhat closer to the free edge. Both openings were irregularly oval in shape and the upper median one was approximately one-sixth of an inch, the lower lateral one-quarter of an inch in diameter.

The latter appeared as though it had originated on the laryngeal surface, the opening at this point being round and smooth while on the lingual side it opened out in a funnel shape, made a deep groove and extended slightly into the base of the tongue. The original point of ulceration in the second opening could not be determined although owing to the greater spreading of the lips on the tongue side it seems probable that it started there. Within the canals could be seen the ragged edges of the necrotic cartilage. (Plate VII, Fig. 26.)

The probability of a syphilitic taint could be almost definitely eliminated, and there were other well marked signs of tuberculosis both in the lungs and larynx.

The entire epiglottis was amputated and numerous sections, embracing both the edges of the perforations and the infiltrated free edge, showed typical tuberculous changes.

Tuberculous perforations of the palate, the only analogous condition, are extremely rare, not more than fifteen cases having been reported, and one of the diagnostic features rests upon the fact that they are always single in contradistinction to the common multiple openings of syphilis, so this case is doubly unique, first, because of the organ affected, and secondly, on account of the openings being two in number.

Ventricular Bands: Isolated ulceration of the ventricular bands is comparatively rare. There is usually simultaneous involvement of other segments of the larynx and there is likewise a strong tendency to spread and involve contiguous tissue.

All forms of ulceration occur but most frequently there is seen the flat, round, superficial, diffuse variety with white base, that bears a striking resemb-

PLATE VII.

Fig. 25.   Ulceration of the lingual surface of the epiglottis and base of the tongue.

Fig. 26.   Double perforation of a greatly infiltrated epiglottis (Dr. Carmody's case).

Fig. 27.   Extensive ulceration of both ventricular bands.

PLATE VII.

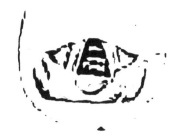

Fig. 25.

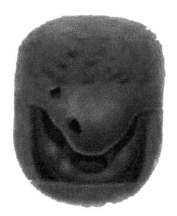

Fig. 26.

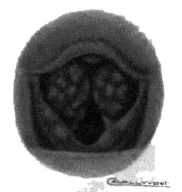

Fig. 27.

PLATE VII.

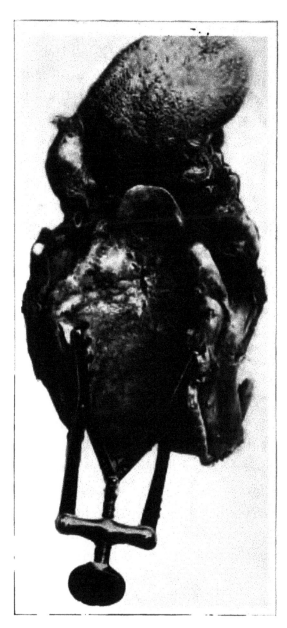

Fig. 28.

lance to the necrosis of diphtheria or that due to concentrated silver solutions. (Plate VII, Fig. 27.)

Frequently the bands are dotted with small round ulcers giving the parts the so-called "sieve" appearance; confluence of these leads to the formation of a single flat, round or irregular ulcer that involves the entire band or a considerable portion thereof.

Because of the large amount of loose submucous tissue severe swelling always accompanies deep ulceration, and the latter may be completely hidden by the protruding mucosa and granulations. (Fig. 28.)

I have seen only one case in which ulcerations of the band were unaccompanied by other evidences of the disease.

Occasionally the anterior wall of the larynx is covered with minute ulcers that are easily overlooked because of the overhang of the epiglottis.

Arytenoids and Aryepiglottic Folds: Ulceration of the aryteno-epiglottidean folds usually occurs late in the course of the disease and is generally superficial; on the arytenoids, particularly the inner surfaces, ulceration is both frequent and early. In the former situation the ulcers are generally superficial, flat and of great size. (See Fig. 21.)

On the arytenoids, in addition to the part already mentioned, they appear on the summit, base and sides, and frequently lead to perichondritis and chondritis. The favored site is the point of convergence of the cord, arytenoid, ventricular band and interarytenoid sulcus.

In many cases the cartilages and folds are converted into large irregular fungous-like bodies through the presence of numerous ulcers and granulations with their attendant edema, that bear but slight resemblance to the normal structures. (Plate VIII, Fig. 29.)

Subglottic   Ulceration: Subchordal ulceration is comparatively rare and of late development. Jurasz has described a form pathognomonic of tuberculosis. It consists of a deep ulcerated groove running parallel with and inferior to the true cord that forms, as it extends, a sort of pocket resembling an artificial subchordal Ventriculus Morgagni.

The cord is apparently thrown into two folds, the upper one the true cord, the lower the linear subchordal mucosa below the pocket.

Ulceration may extend about the entire lumen of the larynx imediately beneath the cords forming a perfect ring.

Both infiltration and ulceration in the subglottic region are clinically rare—(in 3,994 lesions of the larynx, involvement of this region was found only 55 times)—but they are frequently found post mortem.

Tracheal ulceration, in combination with the various laryngeal lesions, is occasionally seen. (Plate VIII, Fig. 30.)

CONDITIONS SECONDARY TO ULCERATION AND INFILTRATION.

Perichondritis is a common sequela of ulceration or extensive infiltration and involves the arytenoids more frequently than all the other cartilages combined. Involvement of these cartilages can usually be attributed to ulcerative processes of the vocal processes, the arytenoidal mucosa, the posterior wall and more rarely the sinus pyriformis.

On the vocal processes especially the cartilage is superficial and exposed, so ulceration readily spreads to and involves the perichondrium.

Laryngoscopic examination rarely gives an exact conception of the existing conditions for uncomplicated perichondrial inflammation offers few distinctive signs; it often simulates infiltration to such an extent that it is impossible to distinguish between them.

Swelling of the cartilage in connection with edema of the aryepiglottic fold is the most frequent manifestation, but cannot be considered distinctive as it also occurs in cases of simple infiltration.

Likewise an edematous swelling of the cartilage, commonly considered pathognomonic, may occur independently of perichondrial involvement and is only strongly suggestive when due to ulceration. '

The most valuable single sign is fixation of the crico-arytenoidal joint; immobility alone, however, is in no way distinctive for it may be the result of simple infiltration of the arytenoidal mucosa.

The coexistence of several of these symptoms, i. e., sudden painful swelling of the cartilage, fixation and edema of the aryepiglottic folds or ventricular bands, either one-sided or bilateral, definitely establishes the diagnosis.

When the process has advanced to the stage of necrosis and abscess formation the diagnosis offers few difficulties.

The abscess opens either near the cartilage of Santorini or at the vocal process and pus exudes upon pressure or during phonation and deglutition.

Through the opening the ragged, necrotic cartilage is sometimes seen and small or large fragments may be thrown off with the pus.

The separation and expulsion of the pieces of cartilage, if considerable fragments are detached, may produce death through asphyxiation; on the other hand, expulsion has taken place without any subjective symptoms.

Subsequent examination shows a marked depression in the region of Santorini's cartilage.

Perichondritis of the cricoid is rare and as a rule involves only one-half the cartilage.

It is usually found in association with perichondritis of the corresponding arytenoid and depends upon the same cause, ulceration of the posterior wall and posterior ends of the vocal cords or of the arytenoids.

Certain exceptional cases may be traced to non-ulcerative infiltrations of the cartilage.

Almost typical of cricoid involvement is the long, narrow, glazed subchordal tumor extending beyond the free edge of the cord, particularly if associated with swelling of the corresponding arytenoid.

Ankylosis of the crico-arytenoidal joint, due to separation of the crico-arytenoideus or to necrosis, and edema of the ventricular bands, ventricles or true cords, are common sequelae and help to differentiate the condition from subchordal infiltration.

When suppuration has occured respiratory fluctuation may be noted, the tumor increasing in size during inspiration and receding with expiration.

Rupture occurs either at the vocal process or at the under side of the cord, and expulsion of large pieces of necrotic cartilage may subsequently occur with sinking of the superimposed parts.

In rare instances the pus follows the ring portion and discharges into the front of the throat or into the trachea.

Perichondritis of the epiglottis almost invariably follows ulceration and in the early stages is not to be distinguished from uncomplicated infiltration.

Tuberculous epiglottic perichondritis never leads to abscess formation and in consequence only molecular necrosis is met; the formation of large sequestra never occurs.

The process is essentially chronic and is marked by a considerable increase in thickness, the epiglottis often reaching to the ventricular bands, the pharyngo- and aryepiglottic folds and the arytenoid cartilages. In the ulcerated areas the ragged edge of the cartilage is often visible. (See Fig. 21.)

Thyroid perichondritis is very rare and almost always results from deep ulcers of the ventricular bands or anterior commissure, although in extremely rare instances it may apparently be the first and only laryngeal focus.

When the inner side is involved examination shows immense swelling of the entire half of the larynx with immobility of the corresponding vocal cord. The swelling usually extends to the subglottic region in the vicinity of the anterior commissure. (Plate IX, Fig. 31.)

When suppuration ensues pointing of the abscess and rupture occur either above or below the commissure or in the anterior part of the ventricle. The in-

PLATE VIII.

Fig. 29.   Ulceration and infiltration of the upper aperture of the larynx. The arytenoid cartilages are converted into a fungoid mass, and the edge of the epiglottis shows several points of ulceration.

Fig. 30.   Tuberculous ulceration of the trachea.

PLATE VIII.

Fig. 29. Ulceration and infiltration of the upper aperture

of the larynx.

Fig. 30. Tuberculous ulceration of the trachea

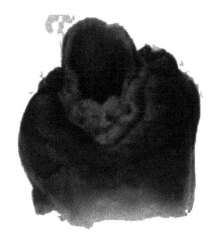

Fig. 29.

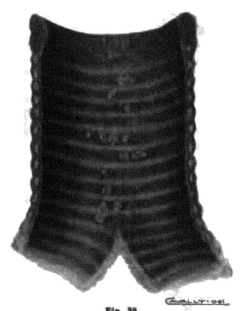

Fig. 30.

flammation may extend through the cartilage and involve the outer plate with the formation of a circumscribed or diffuse fluctuating tumor beneath the skin.

External pressure causes pus to exude into the larynx although this may also happen when the inner plate alone is diseased. Rupture may be followed by the formation of a fistula through which a probe will pass from the skin surface into the interior of the larynx.

Adhesions: The formation of bands of cicatricial tissue, as a result of tuberculous ulceration, is exceedingly rare and few observers have noted its occurrence. Moritz Schmidt has described several cases in which bands of connective tissue formed between the posterior ends of the vocal cords and the posterior wall without, however, extending sufficiently to cause any interference with respiration.

Rosenheim of Baltimore (Laryngoscope, September, 1906), recorded a case in which the tuberculous tissue formed a web between the anterior two-thirds of the cords. In addition to the web there was marked infiltration of both arytenoids and ventricular bands, and the vocal cords were slightly infiltrated and injected. The web was of a reddish color and firm on palpation. Microscopic examination of tissue removed from the arytenoid, as well as from the web, showed typical tuberculous changes.

I have seen one remarkable case of this kind through the courtesy of Dr. T. E. Carmody. The patient, a woman of thirty-four years, had had throat trouble of nearly two years' duration. At the time of her first examination there was tuberculous ulceration of the cords at the anterior commissure, of the left ventricular band, interarytenoid sulcus and left subglottic space. She disappeared for one year when examination showed the following conditions:

The vocal cords are united by two webs, one occupying the anterior one-fourth of the cords, the other the posterior one-third. The posterior web is attached firmly to the posterior wall. The middle third of the left cord is drawn down by adhesions until it occupies a lower plane than the extremities and the opposite cord. (Plate IX, Fig. 32.)

The webs are firm in texture and reddish white in color. The picture is typical of syphilitic disease but there is an absence of any other signs of specific trouble: there are no enlarged glands or other scar tissue; she has had two healthy children and denies all history of syphilis. Specific treatment has had no effect. On the other hand, there is advanced tuberculosis of both lungs, bacilli are constantly present in the sputum and microscopic examination of tissue removed from the larynx shows typical tuberculous changes. There has been considerable dyspnea for the past six months. Despite the clinical history and microscopic findings, one is inclined to consider the case one of mixed infection.

3. THE TUMOR.

Whether or not tuberculous tumors of the larynx are to be looked upon as an extremely rare, or merely a relatively uncommon manifestation of phthisis, depends upon the interpretation of the term tuberculoma.

If the name is limited to those tumor-like growths characterized by absence of bacilli, giant cells and tubercles, then even the most experienced laryngologist will rarely have seen a single example. If, however, the term be accepted in its wider significance as including all growths resembling true tumors, where preceding ulcerations can be definitely eliminated, their comparatively frequent occurrence must be admitted.

The laryngeal tuberculoma is usually secondary but may precede any demonstrable pulmonary lesion: it is sometimes the only laryngeal focus and shows a marked predilection for individuals of an age considerably younger than that at which other tuberculous lesions most commonly occur.

They attack all parts of the larynx but not to an equal extent, and are most common in the ventricles, upon the posterior wall and under the angle of the glottis. Very rarely they occur upon the epiglottis, the ventricular bands and vocal cords.

Panzer (*Wien, Med. Wochen., Nr.* 3-5, 1895), has described three cases of tuberculous polypi in the latter region.

The diagnosis is usually difficult and when unaccompanied by other local or general signs of the disease often impossible without microscopic examination of excised portions of the growth.

In shape they may be round, oval, oblong, lobulated or pedunculated, and in color vary from reddish gray to yellow. They may exist singly or in clusters, in size vary from a pin's head to a cherry or hickory-nut, and in texture be friable or firm and tough. The overlying mucosa is always normal and the surface may be either warty or smooth. The development is very slow. (Plate IX, Fig. 33.)

A common source of error in diagnosis is the mistaking of such conditions as sharply circumscribed infiltrates, prominent granulations, tumors, gummata, lupus, &c., for true tumors.

Trautmann (*Archiv. für Laryngologie,* Bd. XII, 1902) has grouped these widely differing types into the following classes:

(1). "Type d'Avellis," which resembles true fibromata.

(2). "Phthisis pseudo-polypeuse" of Gouguenheim and Tissier.

(3). Recurrent tumors of slow growth, unaccompanied by ulceration and characterized by absence of bacilli, giant cells or tubercles.

To these groups should be added another, including the warty growths of the interarytenoid sulcus, for in many instances they conform perfectly to the conditions generally considered essential.

4. THE MILIARY TUBERCLE.

Miliary tuberculosis of the larynx is so rare that even its occasional occurrence has been denied by many observers.

Undoubtedly many cases so recorded are not examples of miliary tubercles at all, but minute superficial abscesses, obstructed glands, transparent lymph follicles (Schnitzler) and small pale granulations.

That true miliary tubercles are occasionally seen, however, can no longer be doubted although they must be classed as the most infrequent form of laryngeal phthisis.

PLATE IX.

Fig. 31. Perichondritis of the right half of the thyroid cartilage.

Fig. 32. Extensive cicatrization and web formation, due to mixed tuberculosis and syphilis.

Fig. 33. Tuberculoma of the anterior commissure.

PLATE IX.

Fig. 31.   Thyroid parenchymates.

Fig. 32.   Scar tissue due to mixed tuberculosis **and** syphilis.

Fig. 33.   Large gumma at the anterior commissure.

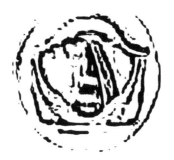

Fig. 31.

Fig. 32.

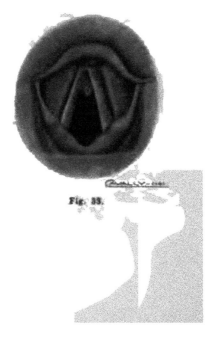

Fig. 33.

Two factors contribute to the rarity of their clinical recognition: their identity is soon lost by conversion into ulcers or they promptly disappear through absorption.

When present they appear as minute gray or yellow nodules upon the base or around the edges of ulcers, over infiltrated areas or upon projecting granulations. According to Moritz Schmidt, they frequently become prominent during treatment by tuberculin.

The possibility of clinically recognizing miliary tubercles has been denied by Heinze on the ground that they are invisible to the naked eye even when fresh ulcerations are removed and examined post mortem.

On the other hand Moritz Schmidt reports a case of extensive ulceration of the ventricular band due to the breaking down of some twenty miliary nodules, and Ph. Schech has described cases of infiltration of the false cords where the miliary nodules were so numerous that they resembled grains of sand thickly sprinkled over the mucosa.

Clinical and anatomical examination showed them to be tubercle conglomerations that later ulcerated and left numerous small apertures resembling a sieve.

Angelot, Orth and Catti (*Wein, Klin. Wochen.*, 1894) have reported cases of acute miliary tuberculosis beginning in the larynx and pharynx.

Catti says the laryngeal symptoms may be so severe as to simulate diphtheria and effectually mask the general symptoms.

The author has seen several cases so distinctive that no doubt could attach to the diagnosis. (Plate XVI, Fig. 51).

One of these, a railroad traffic agent of 34 years, with consolidation of the right upper lobe and bilateral arytenoidal infiltration, developed sudden severe pain in the larynx with a rise of temperature from normal to 102°. The infiltrated arytenoid cartilages showed innumerable minute white spots with intense congestion of the surrounding mucosa. The larynx had been examined a few days before and showed nothing of this nature. Within a few days the nodules over the right cartilage ulcerated and those on the left disappeared. In six weeks the ulcer healed.

A second case occurred in a young electrical engineer, 24 years of age. When first seen there had been hoarseness for one month and severe dysphagia for four days. Examination showed numerous miliary tubercles of the left ventricular band which was chronically infiltrated. The posterior ends of both cords were ulcerated and the left arytenoid was moderately enlarged and covered by miliary tubercles. Temperature 104 1-2, pulse 130. There was slight consolidation of the right upper lobe and the general condition was excellent.

Within thirteen days all the spots had disappeared and both the pulmonary and laryngeal disease improved steadily for five months, when he suffered from a severe attack of ptomain poisoning. Again there was an eruption of miliary tubercles on both arytenoids but the band was not invaded. The attack was ushered in by chills, dysphagia and high temperature.

The pulmonary condition was so aggravated that he went home to New York to die;—eighteen months later he was still living and there had been no recurrence of pain or fever, with the exception of one somewhat similar attack which occurred some ten weeks after the second outbreak, while he was a patient of the Agnes Memorial Sanatorium.

CHAPTER VIII.

DIAGNOSIS.

The diagnosis of laryngeal tuberculosis is simple in typical cases but in certain incipient lesions, atypical cases without constitutional or demonstrable pulmonary manifestations, and uncommon mixed types, syphilis or carcinoma and tuberculosis, it may be exceedingly difficult and at times entirely impracticable.

Primarily it must be understood that neither the tuberculous infiltrate nor ulcer has any absolutely distinctive characteristics aside from the presence of miliary tubercles; certain types may be almost pathognomonic, but atypical lesions of other diseases occasionally show the same peculiarities and invade the same structures.

For example, pear shaped swellings of the arytenoids are usually considered pathognomonic of tuberculosis, yet a corresponding appearance is sometimes given by a unilateral gumma or bilateral edema in nephritis.

The turban-shaped epiglottis may depend upon infectious edema or the perichondritis of syphilis, and uneven projections of the interarytenoid sulcus are occasionally caused by epithelioma, pachydermia, chronic catarrhal laryngitis and certain rare new growths.

In considering the symptomatology it was shown that there is nothing distinctive in the color of the mucous membranes.

Anemia is not characteristic as it occurs in only a small percentage of the cases, is usually a manifestation of general anemia and occurs frequently in otherwise healthy individuals.

The presence of local anemia should suggest the necessity of a thorough general examination, and it may thus lead to the discovery of an otherwise unsuspected tuberculosis, but apart from this it has little diagnostic significance.

When the tuberculous process is fairly well established the diagnosis is easily made even when the lungs are apparently normal.

It is in the incipient stages that the chief difficulties are encountered.

The most typical of the early lesions is infiltration of the interarytenoid sulcus, associated with, or independent of congestion of the vocal cords, and when found in a patient with pulmonary tuberculosis may be considered pathognomonic.

When it occurs in an otherwise apparently normal individual, four conditions must be taken into consideration:—

1. Simple catarrhal hypertrophy.
2. New growths.
3. Pachydermia.
4. Syphilis.

1. The thickening of simple acute or chronic catarrh is generally less extensive, does not show the same marked convexity during phonation, is less translucent

in appearance and is usually smooth in contrast to the rougher and more uneven infiltrate of tuberculosis.

Variations from the typical may occur in either condition, however, through which the types become similar.

In such instances cauterization will frequently clear the diagnosis for it produces prompt recession of the non-tuberculous exudates.

2. New growths of the posterior wall are extremely rare and can only be differentiated from the fullness of tuberculosis by microscopic examination of the excised tissue.

3. When pachydermia is limited to the interarytenoidal mucosa and shows irregular outgrowths, microscopic examination alone can show the true nature of the process.

4. Syphilitic infiltration of the posterior wall may give a picture identical with that due to tuberculosis and the diagnosis must depend upon the history, the further course of the disease and the therapeutic test. It is extremely rare, however, for any of these diseases to be limited to the sulcus without associated lesions of other structures.

CHRONIC CATARRHAL LARYNGITIS.

Incipient tuberculous lesions, if limited to the vocal cords, bear a striking resemblance to the congestion of simple catarrh.

A large percentage of phthisical patients show some evidence of catarrhal laryngitis and the question whether this hyperemia is simple in nature or the result of a submucous infiltrate is hard to answer.

The tuberculous variety rarely involves the entire larynx, or both sides to an equal degree, in contradistinction to catarrhal laryngitis which is practically always universal or symmetrical.

Monochorditis, or an inflammation or thickening of one ventricular band or one-half the epiglottis, never occurs in the simple form and indicates tuberculosis, syphilis, a malignant growth or traumatism.

If the unilateral hyperemia is associated with pulmonary phthisis, and particularly of the corresponding side, the diagnosis is clinched.

The subjective symptoms may aid in determining the true condition, for when we have to deal with an early infiltrate the hoarseness and cough are usually more severe than when dependent upon simple inflammations, owing to the fact that the tuberculous infiltrate begins in the submucous tissues and is more extensive than the changes resulting from simple catarrh.

Early paralysis points to tuberculosis, for it has been shown that this symptom is a comparatively frequent phenomenon even before any laryngeal changes are evident. In this contingency early malignant diseases must also be given consideration, for paralysis or impaired mobility is one of the most suggestive signs of carcinoma.

Simple catarrh is responsive to treatment, hence an unduly intractable case, or one that frequently recurs without obvious cause, is suspicious.

Superficial erosions are found in catarrhal laryngitis but true ulcers never occur.

PACHYDERMIA.

Many cases of pachydermia closely resemble tuberculosis, hence the differential diagnosis is often difficult.

In pachydermia involving the vocal processes the picture is pathognomonic: upon one cord there is a broadbased circumscribed excrescence, upon the corresponding point of the oposite cord a depression into which the excrescence fits. (Plate X, Fig. 34).

Tuberculosis shows no similar appearance. In some instances there is a groove formed in an infiltrated cord by pressure of the opposite one, or an apparent grooving along the free edge due to infiltration of both the superior and inferior surfaces without involvement of the free border, but the conditions are entirely different and the wider involvement in the tuberculous cases is distinctive.

The only condition apparently similar is where one vocal process is deeply ulcerated, forming a triangular pouch, and the other shows circumscribed infiltration at a corresponding point.

Close inspection, however, shows the true condition and in pachydermia true ulceration does not occur. The voice, in tuberculous lesions of this nature, is markedly aphonic; in pachydermia it may be almost normal.

In pachydermia the cords remain freely movable, in tuberculosis there is not infrequently impaired mobility or actual paralysis.

SYPHILIS.

Considerable import has been credited to the site of the lesion in the differentiation of syphilis and tuberculosis.

While each of the diseases has favored points of attack the exceptions are so numerous that they invalidate all diagnostic conclusions based solely upon the regions involved.

Tuberculous ulcers of the epiglottis are usually limited to the tip and laryngeal surface, while syphilis shows a marked predilection for the free edge and the lingual surface.

Although ulceration limited to the lingual surface is highly suggestive of syphilis, tuberculosis rarely attacking this portion, it cannot therefore be inferred that limitation to the under surface and base implies tuberculosis.

I have seen several cases of epiglottic tuberculosis in which the lesions occupied the lingual surface.

Complete destruction of the epiglottis is unquestionably more common in syphilis than in phthisis, but as it does occasionally occur in the latter condition, independent of any other laryngeal focus, its diagnostic worth is almost nil.

Both diseases produce hyperplasia of the inter-arytenoidal mucosa, and in both the lesions are sometimes limited to the vocal cords.

Syphilis attacks the anterior half of the cord more frequently than tuberculosis but isolated ulcers due to the latter condition are occasionally seen about the anterior commissure.

In arriving at a diagnosis, therefore, it is not advisable to give much weight to the site of the lesion.

A single exception, perhaps, can be made in favor of those ulcers limited to the lingual surface of the epiglottis where the probabilities are all in favor of syphilis.

Theoretically, the syphilitic and tuberculous ulcers have certain well marked characteristics, but in practice it is often impossible to distinguish between them.

The ulcer of phthisis is essentially slow in development and occurs in tissues already considerably infiltrated, the margins are ill-defined, merge gradually into the surrounding parts, are wavy and "mouse eaten." If the ulcer is of the deep variety there will be some undermining of the edges.

The edges and base show numerous granulations and are covered by a copious muco-purulent secretion. Scar tissue is rarely seen for there is slight tendency towards spontaneous healing, and the ulcer is usually superficial and has a decided grayish, soft appearance.

The ulcer due to syphilis is of rapid development and is not preceded by chronic infiltration, although there is often considerable edema. It is clear cut, with edges sharply defined, elevated, undermined and prominent, and is usually deep from the outset.

Surrounding it there is a vivid red or purplish areola and the base seldom shows any granulations. (Plate X, Fig. 35.)

Scar tissue often exists in the immediate vicinity and the secretions are more tenacious but less copious than in tuberculosis. The syphilitic ulcer occasions much less pain than the tuberculous.

The one absolutely pathognomonic sign is the presence about the tuberculous ulcer of the numerous small yellow nodules known as miliary tubercles but these are not always present or discernible.

PLATE X.

FIG. 34.   Pachydermia laryngis.

FIG. 35.   Syphilitic ulceration of the larynx.

FIG. 36.   Incipient epithelioma of the vocal cord.

PLATE X.

FIG. 34. Pachydermia laryngis.

FIG. 35. Syphilitic ulceration of the larynx

FIG. 36. Epithelioma of the vocal cord.

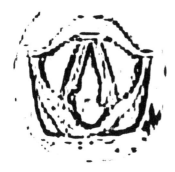

Fig. 34.

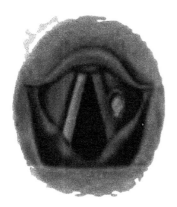

Fig. 35.

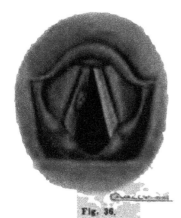

Fig. 36.

The character of the voice is of little assistance for while the syphilitic voice is raucous in contrast with the weak, suppressed voice of phthisis, so many variations occur in each as to destroy any value it might otherwise have.

In all doubtful cases recourse must be had to painstaking general and microscopic examination and the therapeutic test.

In syphilis some other indications of the disease will nearly always be uncovered: ulcers or old scars or swellings of the testicles, penis, lymph glands, palate, pharynx, mouth or bones; skin eruptions, or a history of habitual abortions, &c.

In looking for old signs of syphilis the fact must not be overlooked that in a few well authenticated instances tuberculosis has produced palatal perforation and that when this has occurred the wound has born a striking resemblance to that caused by syphilis.

The same statement holds true in regard to the nasal septum; perforations of the quadrangular cartilage due to tuberculosis are not uncommon, and must be differentiated from simple perforating ulcers and those due to syphilis.

The presence of pulmonary lesions will usually point to tuberculosis but the possibility of a laryngeal syphilis and pulmonary tuberculosis, or laryngeal tuberculosis and syphilis of the lungs, must not be overlooked.

Both diseases are occasionally present in the larynx at the same time.

The therapeutic test will usually promptly clear the diagnosis but one element of doubt may arise within the first few weeks. It occasionally happens that even the tuberculous lesions will improve temporarily under such treatment, but it is always fleeting and, the lesions promptly lose all they have gained. ·

The same phenomenon is occasionally observed in malignant growths, due to temporary absorption of the surrounding inflammatory edema.

In all doubtful cases examination should be made of portions of the involved tissues and of secretions from the ulcer, but even in typical tuberculous ulcers examination may fail to demonstrate bacilli, tubercles or giant cells, for it is often impossible to remove more than the surface and hence a negative result is valueless.

Bacilli are always present in the secretions of tuberculous laryngeal ulcers and an attempt may be made to demonstrate them.

The larynx should be thoroughly cleansed by antiseptic sprays and swabs, and the ulcer touched by a cotton-wound applicator.

If tubercle bacilli are found it is practically diagnostic, although it must be admitted that, despite the careful local cleansing, they may have been deposited by the sputum.

A diagnosis by means of tuberculin injections is often possible and is unattended by danger.

If the local condition is tuberculous an increase in the hyperemia, with a marked rise of temperature within one to two hours, will usually follow the injection of one milligram. Miliary tubercules sometimes appear over the infiltrated tissues.

If no reaction occurs, a larger dose may be given after one or two days, and if still without result, a yet larger injection—10 milligrams—after another two days.

Tuberculosis can be almost definitely excluded if no reaction then occurs.

PROLAPSE OF THE VENTRICLE.

Prolapse of the ventricle may be mistaken for tuberculosis when the inferior part of the ventricle is infiltrated to such an extent that it partially overhangs the vocal cord. Firm pressure with a cotton-tipped applicator will cause recession of the prolapse.

LUPUS.

Laryngeal lupus is almost always secondary to disease of the skin and neighboring mucous membranes and is then easily recognized.

When the laryngeal deposit is primary it bears a strong resemblance to tuberculosis and might readily be mistaken for it.

The nodules of lupus are extremely indolent and ulcerate so slowly that one part cicatrizes while another is disintegrating; thus infiltration, ulceration and cicatrization are found side by side.

Lupus is extremely rare, runs an almost painless course and is frequently limited to the epiglottis.

LEPROSY.

Leprosy is never limited to the larynx and the skin condition is pathognomonic.

Hoarseness and dyspnea are always present but dysphagia has not occurred in the few cases observed.

The epiglottis is usually thickened and edematous, ulceration may be absent or occur only late in the disease, the mucous membrane is hyperemic and the tubercles, when present, appear as rounded nodules with a skin-like surface. The condition is extremely rare.

CARCINOMA.

Carcinoma in the pre-ulcerative stages, or in rarer instances where there is beginning ulceration of the diffuse infiltrative type, closely simulates tuberculosis.

Particularly is this the case where the lungs are apparently normal and the individual past the meridian of life.

If the growth is of the typical fungus variety or if marked ulceration or lymphatic involvement has occurred, no difficulty in differentiation is encountered, but if it appears as a smooth, diffuse infiltrate, microscopic examination alone will reveal the true nature.

Carcinomatous growths of this type have been frequently observed and are usually situated in the ventricle or upon the ventricular bands,—a common site of the tuberculous infiltrate. It is rare, however, for the latter condition to be strictly isolated, there being practically always simultaneous involvement of the cords or interarytenoid incisure.

The malignant growth, on the other hand, usually occurs in a larynx otherwise normal, except perhaps for a chronic laryngitis.

Epithelioma of the vocal cords, in the still curative stages, is likewise of doubtful appearance and might occasionally be mistaken for phthisis. (Plate X, Fig. 36.)

On the cords it appears as a warty growth, as a diffuse infiltration or as a monochorditis. The warty form bears some resemblance to a tuberculoma but the latter usually lacks the inflamed base of the malignant growth and is not so apt to cause impaired mobility.

Ph. Shech reports a case in which one-half the larynx was removed because of a circumscribed, broad-based, warty excrescence upon the left cord that was apparently of a malignant nature. Examination of the excised tumor proved it to be tuberculous.

Neither of the other conditions, i. e., diffuse infiltration or monochorditis, offers any distinctive signs. A dirty white opaque appearance is suggestive of malignancy and likewise an early loss of mobility of the involved cord.

Too much importance should not be attached to this early paralysis, however, for while it undoubtedly occurs in nearly all cases of malignancy, it has been shown to be a comparatively frequent symptom of early tuberculosis as well.

The subjective symptoms are similar in the two diseases. The character of the pain provoked is not distinctive. De Santi (Malignant Disease of the Larynx, p. 36) claims that the radiating pains to the ear are very characteristic of malignancy in that they are not so frequently noted in other affections of the larynx.

We have seen, however, in considering the subjective symptoms, that this aural pain is a frequent accompaniment of tuberculous disease and is present in practically all the dysphagic cases.

The age of the individual is of little real service in differentiation. Milignancy is rare before the fortieth year, yet in 588 cases, nine occurred between the tenth and twentieth years, thirty between 20 and 30 and fifty-eight beween 30 and 40.

In 2542 cases of tuberculosis, 404 occurred in individuals over 40 years of age.

Thus, while tuberculosis is most common before 40 and carcinoma after this age, the exceptions are so frequent as to destroy its worth except as a suggestive sign, for of the carcinomatous cases 16.5 per cent occurred in individuals under forty years of age and of the tuberculous, 15.8 per cent in those over forty.

The absence or presence of glandular enlargement is not often of practical assistance.

Krishaber's statement that "as long as the cancer remains intrinsic there is no cervical glandular enlargement; when it is extrinsic the glands are infected;"—has been well substantiated, but in a not inconsiderable percentage of tuberculous cases there is more or less extensive involvement of the cervical and sub-maxillary glands, occurring without relation to the extent or locale of the lesions.

In all doubtful cases a considerable fragment should be excised, cutting well into the base, and examined microscopically for the characteristic features of both conditions.

CHAPTER IX.

PROGNOSIS.

In tuberculosis a definite prognosis is seldom permissible and to the larynx this rule applies with even greater force than to the lungs. So many factors are to be considered aside from the extent and locale of the laryngeal process, i. e., pulmonic or other organic tuberculosis, occurrence of intercurrent diseases, constitutional idiosyncrasies and weaknesses, the social and financial status, the moral and physical fortitude, &c., that anything more than a tentative prognosis is equally unwise and unwarranted.

A decade ago the advent of laryngeal tuberculosis was considered as rendering the prognosis invariably hopeless, while even to-day the view of a recent authority that "occasionally a case recovers; nearly all die," is almost universally accepted. That this is the commonly accepted dictum is shown by the following citations:

"We can hardly hope to do much more than retard its progress, and thereby prolong for a few months the life of the patient."—*Sajous.*

"The prognosis is always extremely grave, and it is not certain that any case recovers."—*Sir Morell MacKenzie*, 1880.

"As to figures, we might quote from John N. Mac-Kenzie, who deduced the fact that in 100 cases death resulted in from twelve to eighteen months after the usual symptoms showed themselves, and that in 6 per cent a fatal issue occurred within six months."

"Bosworth gives forty-six months as the longest time, and three months as the shortest time, after pulmonary tuberculosis was complicated with laryngeal invasion, or to quote his summary:—

"The average duration of life in an ordinary attack of pulmonary consumption is three years; the average duration of life in an attack of pulmonary consumption complicated by laryngeal invasion is eighteen months."—*Jonathan Wright*, 1902.

Dr. Ph. Schech (*Handbuch der Laryngologie*), in summarizing his views, says:

"Nevertheless, as even M. Schmidt and Heryng, the most outspoken advocates of the curability of laryngeal phthisis, agree, the number of complete and lasting cures is very small. Generally there is a recurrence after a shorter or longer time, and this is usually severer and more widespread than the primary attack: or the lung process makes such progress that the fatal result will be hastened thereby."

Dr. W. C. Phillip of New York, in 1906, said that he had never seen a case involving the vocal cords, the epiglottis, the false cords and the arytenoids, recover. In his opinion they are always fatal.

"When extensive ulceration of the larynx is found, we may safely predict that the patient will not live more than eight or twelve weeks. A few cases die within six weeks of the beginning of the disease. It is not the belief, as formerly, that all of these cases are fatal, for there is ample proof that a few recover. We nearly always find accompanying pulmonary tuberculosis and it is probably safe to say that where laryngeal tuberculosis is so complicated, nine-tenths of the patients die."—*Ingals, Diseases of the Chest, Throat and Nasal Cavities*, p. 441.

Dr. H. Bert Ellis, of Los Angeles, at the twelfth annual meeting of the American Laryngological, Rhinological and Otological Society, held in Kansas City, Missouri, June, 1906, said that when he sees a case of serious tuberculosis of the larynx with considerable infiltration, he feels tolerably certain that the patient will die within six months to a year. He does not believe in local treatment.

Such pessimism is entirely unjustified for while this form of phthisis must always be looked upon as a most serious one, the disease may be cured in a considerable percentage and temporarily arrested in the majority of all cases.

In no other disease is a statistical report of so little value for we are dealing not with a process of standard or even fairly equable conditions, but with one where each is a law unto itself; yet when we contrast the percentage of recoveries quoted by Bosworth in 1893 (less than 1 per cent) with those by such a conservative authority as Solly, computed from cases treated in Colorado, it is seen that progress has been real and substantial and that this present pessimism is illogical.

Solly says:

"Taking the results in laryngeal cases without considering the ultimate fate of the patient, there was permanent arrest of the disease in 64 per cent; temporary arrest in 5 per cent additional cases in which the tissue again broke down shortly before death. Looking at the ulcerated cases alone, 50 per cent healed permanently, 10 per cent temporarily."

Levy, in 1900, reported 26 deaths in 86 infiltrative cases. Of 60 ulcerative cases 37 grew worse or died, and of those without involvement of the epiglottis or aryepiglottic folds only 10 per cent died or failed to improve.

Lake has compiled the following table:

	No. of Cases	Cures	Improved
Heryng	200	20	
Schmidt	300	16	33
Lake	329	48	
Total	829	84	33

While the contrast between the results in Lake's tabulation, showing about 10 per cent of recoveries, and those of a decade ago is striking, it is not so remarkable as that between this 10 per cent and the approximate 55 per cent of Solly and other Colorado observers. In the second edition of his work, Lake says:

"In the first edition I recorded 48 cures out of 329 cases, or 14.59 per cent; and from 1901 to 1903 inclusive, I have to record, out of 211 cases, 44 cures, or 20.85 per cent, and 14.21 per cent much improved."

Of the earlier reports the most favorable are those of . Schmidt:

Year	Cases	Healed	Percentage
1888 181		34	18.7%
1889 179		30	16.5%
1890 155		32	20.6%
1891 195		36	18.4%
1892 188		39	20.7%
Total 898		171	18.99%

He has classed as "healed" all those remaining well at the end of the year during which they received treatment. Upon this report he makes the following comments:

"A goodly proportion remained well still longer, certain it is that the greater number relapsed the following year."

The majority of these cases were ambulatory and lived under unhygienic conditions and in an unfavorable climate and easily relapsed into the old methods of living after a seeming recovery. The percentage of cures in such cases is naturally much less than among the better class of private and sanatorium patients.

The word "arrest" instead of "cure" should be used in all the above tabulations for the ultimate fate of the pulmonic process is not considered. The great differences in the mortality as detailed in these reports, approximately 40 per cent, probably represents in part the increased chances of improvement during residence in the favored climates,—Lake's, Heryng's and Schmidt's patients being drawn from London, Berlin and Frankfort respectively, while Solly's, Levy's and a majority of the author's cases were observed in Colorado.

This is due not so much to the direct effect of the favored climates upon the throat lesions as to the coin-

cident improvement of the pulmonic process, the ultimate *sine qua non* of prognosis.

In connection with the statement regarding the effects of the so-called favorable climates, it is interesting to note the observation of Thost to the effect that
laryngeal tuberculosis is much rarer and less severe
in the damp climate of Hamburg than in the drier,
dustier atmosphere of Vienna.

A conservative estimate to-day would place the percentage of probable recoveries at between 50 and 60
per cent, without taking into consideration the ultimate fate of the individual, i. e., the pulmonic process,
and each year the outlook grows increasingly bright
notwithstanding the fact that our armamentarium has
few remedies of greater efficacy than it contained a
decade ago.

What is the explanation of this apparent paradox?

It depends in large measure upon earlier recognition of the incipient lesions, more universal ultilization
of the essentials of treatment, local and constitutional,
and to an almost equal degree upon the mental attitude
of the physician and patient.

Convinced of its incurability the laryngologist formerly treated throat tuberculosis in a perfunctory manner, striving after the single goal of euthanasia, while
to-day, with deep appreciation of the necessity of constant vigilance and supervision with its common re-
ward, his increased zeal and confidence bring infinitely
greater success.

Moreover, pulmonary tuberculosis is now much more
widely recognized in its earlier stages, and suitable
treatment, hygienic and climatic, is generally instituted

while there is yet good hope of eventual cure. In consequence, the laryngeal complications are much rarer than formerly and more amenable to treatment when discovered.

In considering the curability of the throat lesions, prime importance must be placed upon the degree of pulmonary involvement and the general condition and powers of resistance, for the outcome of the laryngeal process must always depend in large measure upon the general constitutional state.

That the progress of the laryngeal disease is in keeping with that of the lungs is the common but not invariable rule. This interdependence from a prognostic standpoint is most clearly shown by study of the so-called primary cases (laryngeal without demonstrable or only slight pulmonary or other organic disease) where practically all cases recover.

With each step in the advancement of the lung lesion the arrest of the throat process becomes increasingly difficult. This is due equally to impaired resistance entailing lowered powers of reparation, and to the increased likelihood of reinfection through the medium of sputum, blood or lymph.

With far advanced lesions of the lungs, in miliary tuberculosis and in those cases with persistent hyperpyxeria little can be anticipated beyond temporary control, or in advanced cases, the partial relief of dyspnea and dysphagia, but this end justifies vigorous measures in all cases where such symptoms are to be apprehended.

Even with a rapidly progressing pulmonary lesion where the end can be definitely prognosticated, arrest or complete cure of the throat lesion may not infrequently result. *Per contra*, steady disintegration of the laryngeal structures occasionally accompanies a cicatrizing or already healed lung.

It has been frequently claimed that laryngeal improvement never accompanies advancing pulmonic conditions, but such is entirely contrary to my experience. It is not alone common, but frequent.

The laryngeal lesions associated with fibroid phthisis offer a much more favorable prognosis than those complicating the more acute forms, and the outlook is also more generally favorable in those who have accidentally acquired the disease than in those with bad family and personal history.

In general, it may be said that those symptoms which render doubtful the outcome of the constitutional malady bespeak the same doubt in so far as the throat is concerned.

THE LOCALE OF THE LESION IN ITS PROGNOSTIC SIGNIFICANCE.

The most serious and obstinate of all the lesions of laryngeal tuberculosis are those of the epiglottis. Extensive ulceration or universal infiltration usually warrants an unfavorable prognosis, although even the severest cases may occasionally recover, as is shown by the following statistics in which there is a percentage of 11.95 in arrested cases, and an additional 31.54 per cent in which there was temporary improvement:

EPIGLOTTIS.

	No. Cases.	Arrested	Im- proved.	Unim- proved.	Percentage of Arrested Cases.
Incipient	13	7	4	2	53.84
Moderate	22	8	6	8	36.36
Advanced	92	11	29	52	11.95
Total	127	26	39	62	34.05

In 72 cases of epiglottic disease recorded by Lake, amount of involvement not given, eleven, or one in six and a half cases, died.

Moderate involvement, either in the form of shallow ulcerations or circumscribed infiltrations, is more serious than extensive intrinsic disease.

Owing to the intimate connection between the mucous membrane and the perichondrium, inflammation of the latter almost invariably ensues at an early date with resultant necrosis of the cartilage. In these cases there is usually severe and uncontrollable dysphagia, regurgitation and some dyspnea.

Next in point of danger ranks general involvement of the arytenoids and aryteno-epiglottidean folds. These lesions, as well as those of the epiglottis with which they are often associated, are late manifestations of the disease, originating, as a rule, when both the pulmonary and laryngeal infections are far advanced and progressive.

In consequence of this, as well as because they provoke lasting dysphagia, the prognosis is generally bad.

Isolated ulceration or infiltration of the arytenoid cartilages is fairly responsive to treatment, but when the disease has spread to the aryteno-epiglottidean folds the outlook is much less promising. If at the same time there is epiglottidean involvement, there. is extremely small chance of arrest.

Region.	No. Cases.	Arrests.	Im- proved.	Unim- proved.	Percentage of Arrested Cases.
Epiglottis, Arytenoids and Aryteno-Epiglottidean Folds 73		5	22	46	6.8 %
Arytenoids and Aryteno- Epiglottidean Folds ... 47		12	19	16	25.53%
Arytenoids alone 150		80	44	26	53.33%
Total 270		97	85	88	

Destruction of the various cartilages is of **grave** significance, both because of the local conditions upon which the necrosis depends and because it is usually found in association with progressive pulmonary disease or with general miliary tuberculosis. The arytenoids, however, are sometimes subject to disintegration and the separation of large sequestra without serious results.

Circumscribed ulcerations and infiltrations of the interarytenoid incisure respond well to treatment. Superficial ulcerations of the ventricular bands and vocal cords heal in the majority of all cases, while even extensive disease of these segments, if the remaining tissues are uninvolved, can usually be conquered.

Region.	No. Cases	Arrests.	Im- proved.	Unim- proved.	Percentage of Arrested Cases.
Isolated Lesions of Inter- arytenoid Sulcus....... 79		51	26	2	64.55%
Isolated Lesions of Vocal Cords 21		19	⌀	0	90.47%
Lesions of Ventricular Bands without serious disease of other parts... 9		6	3	0	66.66%
Total 109		76	31	2	

The association of two or more of these processes naturally lessens the chance of improvement, and unfortunately there are usually several distinct foci.

Both the site and extent of the lesions must be considered in arriving at an estimate of the probable chances of recovery, and it is this factor which makes it difficult to draw any conclusions of definite worth from tabulated reports.

In the entire series of cases reported, 506, there were 199 of definite arrest, 39.32 per cent; and 155 additional cases, or 30.63 per cent, in which there was improvement during the period of treatment. There remain 398 cases not covered by this report, in which the lesions were of such character as to render definite classification impracticable.

Classified in the two primary groups of "Infiltrative" and "Ulcerative" cases, we have the following:

Type	No. Cases	Arrests	Percentage of Arrests
Infiltrative Cases 537		326	60.7
Ulcerative Cases 367		194	52.8
Total 904		520	56.75

It is impossible to say what percentage of these arrested cases remain well, for after temporary cure the great majority disappear and are never seen or heard from again. It is certain that a not inconsiderable percentage relapse and that a large number perish from other tuberculous processes, but that enduring cures are frequent, even in those with advanced lesions, regardless of the eventual outcome of the pulmonic process, has been attested by a large number of cases in all sections of the world.

THE VOICE.

Long periods of partial or complete aphonia may be succeeded by normal tone production—normal not only in resonance but in sustained power as well. As a rule, however, the voice remains permanently rough and inflexible.

The most promising cases are those in which the condition is due to functional causes, or to the early infiltrates and superficial ulcerations of the vocal cords and interarytenoid sulcus.

Aphonia consequent upon recurrent paralysis or ankylosis of the crico-arytenoidal articulation is nearly always permanent, although some cases due to the latter condition recover.

Deep ulceration of the cords, causing considerable loss of tissue and the so-called "saw tooth" edge, generally produces permanent hoarseness but perfect restoration is sometimes attained even after widespread and seemingly permanent destruction.

DYSPHAGIA.

The minor degrees of dysphagia are generally amenable to treatment but the more severe cases, due to extensive extrinsic lesions, are exceedingly rebellious. In the great majority of such instances temporary palliation is the *ultima thule* of our endeavors.

The development of dysphagia, in the vast majority of all cases, can be prevented by recognition and treatment of the incipent lesions.

When far advanced, medicinal treatment is mostly ineffectual and radical intralaryngeal surgical management is required.

PLATE XI.

FIG. 37. Case ending in spontaneous cure coincident with rapid progression of the pulmonic process.

FIG. 38. Lesions resulting in spontaneous cure in a patient whose general condition was undergoing speedy improvement.

PLATE XI.

FIG. 37. Case ending in spontaneous cure. .

FIG. 38. Case ending in spontaneous cure.

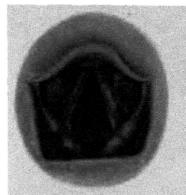

Fig. 37.

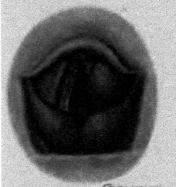

Fig. 38.

DYSPNEA.

Dyspnea rarely advances to the point of threatened asphyxiation. It is usually of slow development and responds to medical and surgical treatment, so it is only in the exceptional cases that tracheotomy is necessitated.

Massier (*Archives Internationales de Laryngologie*, xviii, No. 5, 1904) described a case of death from glottic spasm in a patient with slight laryngeal tuberculosis;—and instances of sudden asphyxiation, due to bilateral abductor paraylsis, are recorded. I have already described such a case (pg. 91).

MILIARY TUBERCULOSIS.

Miliary tuberclosis of the larynx is invariably fatal when a manifestation of general miliary tuberculosis. Localized miliary tubercles, on the other hand, while usually of grave significance, may occasionally cicatrize.

PREGNANCY.

The relationship between the larynx and female genitalia is an intimate one. At puberty, during the period of "change of voice," the laryngeal mucosa is subject to attacks of congestion and similar hyperemic seizures occur during menstruation, pregnancy, &c.

Among normal individuals the influence of this physiologic process is especially evident in singers whose vocal organs are unduly sensitive to all such influences.

Of pathologic conditions none are so susceptible to these same influences as tuberculosis. The swelling and congestion are usually markedly increased during the menstrual periods while pregnancy almost invariably causes rapid and fatal destruction. Of fifteen personal cases reported by Küttner, all but one of whom acquired the disease during pregnancy, all died before or within two months after delivery.

Godskesen has collected 46 additional cases, the results of which may be summarized as follows:

35 treated endolaryngeally.

23 died during pregnancy or within two months after delivery or abortion.

  2 cases of tuberculous tumor; operated; successful delivery.

  8 other cases: successful delivery.

  2 other cases: lost sight of before term.

11 cases treated extra-laryngeally.

  8 tracheotomies.

  3 died immediately after delivery or abortion.

  5 successfully delivered.

  3 cases by laryngofissure and tracheotomy.

  1, five months pregnant, recovered from operation and lost sight of.

  2 other cases: death.

Resume of 25 cases complicating pregnancy, by Küttner (*Annal. des Maladies de l'Oreille et de Larynx,* 1901, XVII):

  3, pulmonary tuberculosis before pregnancy.

12, pulmonary lesions doubtful.

  1, laryngitis preceded conception.

  2, laryngitis appeared in 6th month.

12, laryngitis appeared during first half of pregnancy.

1 with an apical lesion, and one with laryngeal tuberculosis, who had been free from symptoms 3 to 4
years, died after delivery.

None of the cases reached full term.

4 reached the ninth month.

8 reached the eighth month.

3 reached the seventh month.

Eight infants died within three weeks.

Sokolowsky (*Berliner Klinische Wochenschrift,* July
1904) records 71 cases of laryngeal tuberculosis complicated by pregnancy:

14 cases, results unknown.

56 died during or soon after confinement.

1 lived eight years.

One case seen by the author, in which both the mother and child survived, is recorded on pages 171 and 172.

Nearly all the children born of such mothers die in
early infancy. Few women with laryngeal tuberculosis become pregnant owing to the severe anemia
usually accompanying such conditions.

It may be considered axiomatic that pregnancy predisposes to tuberculous laryngitis, and will practically
always cause a recurrence in healed lesions and a
lighting up of incipient or quiescent cases.

That pregnant women with phthisis so frequently
develop laryngeal complications is due to the concomitant increase of the constitutional malady, to the previously considered relationship between the larynx and
genitalia and to the general lessening of vitality, the
anorexia, &c. The same causes explain the rapidity
with which old lesions advance.

If the laryngeal disease is far advanced the outcome is nearly always fatal; if incipient, prompt abortion offers the only fair hope of recovery. If abortion be impossible, tracheotomy should be performed at the earliest possible moment.

Cases	Lost Sight of	Successful Delivery (After Operation)	Died
15...........	0	0	15
35...........	2	10	. *23
8...........	0	5	† 3
3...........	1	0	† 2
61	3	15	43

*Endolaryngeal operations.
†Tracheotomy and Laryngofissure.

Since the above was written, every reported case has been collected and tabulated by Küttner. This table is appended.

(See Table on Opposite Page.)

SYPHILIS.

Next to pregnancy syphilis is the gravest of complicating diseases. If the tuberculous condition is in its incipiency healing may result, but when the lesions are advanced, even if the syphilitic spots can be brought under control, the tuberculosis rapidly advances. Several observers report cases in which the syphilitic complication seemed to exert a favorable influence upon the tuberculosis.

No.	Author	Reference	Report Cases	Recov. Cases / Cures	Favor	Died	Died	Favo
1	Earlier cases collected by A. Kuttner	Berl. klin. Wchschr. 1905, Nr. 29.	cir. 100	cir. 100	3		3	
2	Pradella	Vrhdlg. d. D. laryng. Ges. 1905.	3	3	2			
3	Frischbier	J. D., Basel 1906	5	5				
4	Felix	Annales des maladies de l'oreille, etc. 1906, no. 2	2	2	2			
5	Freudenthal	Ztschr. f. Tuberkulose etc. Bd. XI. Heft 5.	26	26	2		2	
6	Clifton, Edgar	Ibidem.	2	1				
7–8	Marx	Ibidem.	2	2				
8	Lühnberg[1]	Private communication	4	3				
9	Levinger[2]	Münch. med. Wchschr. 1906, Nr. 23	2	2	1			
10	Beta[3]	Private communication	1	1				
11	Reiche	Münch. med. Wchschr. 1905, Nr. 28.	9	9				
12	Cohn-Bromberg	Private communication	9	9				
13	Kuttner, A.	Vrhdlg. d. Berl. laryng. Ges. 1905, 20.	1	1				
14	Jan		1	1				
15	Alexander	Ibidem.	1	1				
16	Ed. Meyer	Ibidem.	1	1				
17	Rosenberg, A.	Ibidem.	2	2				
18	Veit, J.	Therapie d. Gegenwart, 1906, p. 431	3	3				
19	Lennhof	Vrhdlg. d. Berl. laryng. Ges. 1906	1	1				
20	Ch. Parker, H. Tilley, L. Lack, Cl. Beale	Intern. Centralbl. f. Laryngol. etc. 1906, p. 31 u. 32.	4	4				
21	Rosthorn[4]	Mtaschr. f. Geburtsh. u. Gynäk. Bd. 23, p. 581	4	4	1			
22	Jurasz	Ibidem, p. 731	3	2				
23	Koppe	Centralbl. f. Gynäk. 1887, p. 153	37	37				
24	Lomer	Frauenarzt, 1904	1	1				
25	H. W. Freund	Winckels Hdbch. d. Geburtsh. Bd. 2, Tl. I, p. 596.	1	1				
26	Barthes, F.	Thèse de Paris, 1906	4	4	1			
27	J. B. Cragin	s Freudenthal, 1906	14	6				
28	Kollege K.	Ibidem.	1	1				
			240	230	9	3	1	6	4

1. One case not under observation up to the time of confinement.
2. The death of one patient was caused by a tuberculous laryngeal tumor.
3. Of the new cases reported by Betz, four have taken a very favorable course. (Thr... cation.) In three of the new cases the affection of the larynx developed in the eighth and n... the wealthy classes.
4. In the middle of the seventh month.
5. In the third case, also dead, the larynx-diagnosis was doubtful.

INFLUENCE OF AGE.

Either extreme of age, infancy or old age, renders the outlook doubly serious though a few notable cases of recovery at each extreme have been observed. A case is recorded of a man of seventy-four in whom tuberculous laryngitis developed and healed.

PATHOLOGIC FINDINGS.

An attempt has been made to judge of the severity of the process by the peculiar pathologic conditions present in the individual case. (Baumgarten-Heryng).

Thus it is claimed that the severest type is that represented by tissue composed of pure lymphoid-celled tubercles rich in bacilli; the most amenable, the epithelioid or giant cell tubercles with few bacilli, while those composed of lymphoid and epithelioid varieties occupy a medium position.

Such deductions, according to my experience, are absolutely unreliable, no relation whatever existing between the severity of the case and the type of the tissue existent, and in many cases the exact opposite obtains.

Upon the most florid case within the author's remembrance the following report was submitted by the pathologist, Dr. J. A. Wilder:

"Sections from the tissue of the larynx, case of Mr. F., show the general changes of tuberculosis.

"The tubercles show no evidence of caseation and consist chiefly of connective tissue cells and lymphoid cells with a moderate number of epithelioid and giant cells. Numerous sections stained for tubercular bacilli show them to be present in very small numbers only. Three typical bacilli only were found after a prolonged search.''

SPONTANEOUS HEALING.

While it may be stated, as a general rule, that healing occurs only when the pulmonary process improves or becomes quiescent, cases of spontaneous healing have been reported, not alone in quiescent cases but also in those suffering rapid disintegration.

Schech reports a case of complete healing in a patient with extensive laryngeal ulceration whose general condition was rapidly growing worse, and I have seen two such cases.

The most striking of these was a man of twenty-seven years who presented marked ulceration of both cords and the interarytenoid sulcus, with extensive infiltration of the ventricular bands. (Plate XI, Fig. 37.) His general condition was so bad that he was advised to return to his home in the East, where he died seven months later. Shortly before death I had the privilege of examining his larynx and found it entirely healed. No treatment had been given other than a cleansing spray.

The lesions in the second case consisted of infiltration of both arytenoid cartilages, ulceration of the right cord and infiltration of the left ventricular band and sulcus. (Plate XI, Fig. 38.)

Eisenbarth has reported a case of spontaneous cure of the laryngeal disease in a man with both pulmonary and intestinal tuberculosis.

PLATE XII.

PLATE XII.

Figs. 39-40-41. Case showing rapid recurrence of lesions that had been brought to a point of virtual arrest.

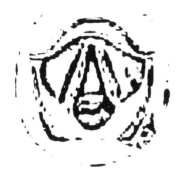

Fig. 39.

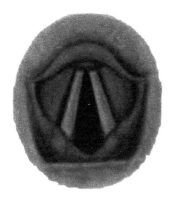

Fig. 40.

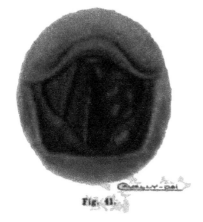

Fig. 41.

PLATE XII.

Heryng reports 14 cases of spontaneous healing in 2810 cases of laryngeal tuberculosis.

The slighter involvements, infiltrations and congestions, and occasionally shallow ulcerations, frequently improve and rarely entirely recover coincident with the improvement of the general condition, but it is unwise to forego local treatment because of this shadowy hope for nearly every case will steadily progress unless energetically handled.

RECURRENCE.

In conclusion, attention is directed to the fact that in speaking of the result, the words "healed" and "arrested" lesions have been advisedly employed.

A cure cannot be claimed until a number of years, from two to five, have elapsed from the time of apparent arrest, and it cannot be gainsaid that these lasting cures are uncommon, owing to steady progression of the process in the lungs.

After varying intervals recurrences are probable and are usually of severer type than the original infection.

The recurrences are generally due to some insult to an incapsulated tubercle long quiescent, and could usually be avoided by a continuance, after an apparent cure, of those hygienic dietetic rules in force during the period of active treatment, but it is only the exceptional person who can continue to hold out against the allurements of city life. If relapse occurs the prognosis is usually worse than in primary attacks. (Plate XII, 39, 40 and 41.)

Laryngeal phthisis, when complicated by invasion

CHAPTER X.

RECORDS.

Showing Possibilities of Treatment in Some Apparently Hopeless Cases.

A small number of case reports are appended, not because they are in any respect typical or indicative of the results usually to be attained, but because they offer a striking exemplification of the idea so frequently reiterated throughout this work, i. e., the occasional curability of even the most advanced cases and the wisdom, therefore, of persistent treatment of every such patient, regardless of the extent, character and locale of the lesions.

CASE I.

W. P. G., a man of twenty-six years, was first seen in June, 1903. He had come to Colorado in January of the same year, nearly twenty-four months after the recognized onset of his pulmonary symptoms, and had been advised because of his extensive pulmonary involvement, emaciation, high temperature and pulse, to at once return home. There was complete aphonia of thirteen months' duration, and for eight weeks he had had severe dysphagia with slowly developing dyspnea.

On examination of the larynx the following picture

presented: enormous swelling of both arytenoids almost closing the laryngeal aperture, which was still
further encroached upon by the edematous aryteno-
epiglottidean folds; moderate infiltration and deep ulceration upon the laryngeal surface of the epiglottis;
vocal cords almost completely hidden. (Plate XIII,
Fig. 42.)

No hope of permanent benefit was held, but for the
relief of the dysphagia the affected part of the epiglottis was removed and ten days later both arytenoids
were cut back as far as possible. Between operations
and subsequently, daily applications of five per cent
formalin were made.

The operations resulted in complete relief of the
dysphagia, and there was rapid improvement in the
general health with an increase in weight of seventeen
pounds within four weeks of the time of healing of
the last operation wound.

Laryngeal improvement was both rapid and continuous, and by February, 1905, twenty months from the
time of first examination, he was pronounced cured
both as to the lungs and larynx. At that time there
had been no dysphagia for over a year and the voice
was practically normal, both in volume and flexibility.

There has been no relapse.

CASE II.

G. P., an accountant, was referred to me in April,
1905. He had lived in Colorado for fifteen years and
had acquired pulmonary tuberculosis while serving in
the army of the Philippines.

The lungs showed consolidation with moist rales on

PLATE XIII.

Fig. 42. Edema of the arytenoid cartilages and aryteno-epiglottidean folds. The epiglottis is thickened and ulcerated. (Case I.)

Fig. 43. Massive infiltration and extensive ulceration of left ventricular band: bilateral arytenoidal ulceration and infiltration: ulceration of the right vocal cord and of the interarytenoid sulcus. (Case II.)

Fig. 44. Ulceration and infiltration of both vocal cords, ragged infiltration of the posterior wall, and perichondritis of the left arytenoid. (Case III.)

right vocal cord and of the interarytenoid sulcus.

FIG. 44. Ulceration and infiltration of both vocal cords, ragged infiltration of the posterior wall, and perichondritis of the left arytenoid.

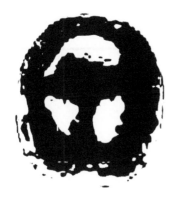

Fig. 42.

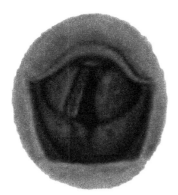

Fig. 43.

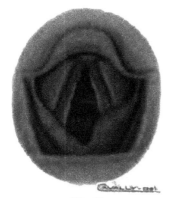

Fig. 44.

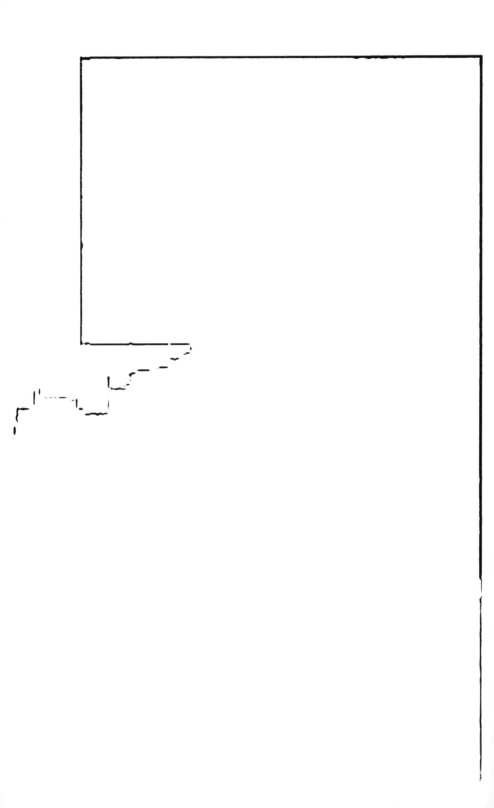

both sides down to the fourth rib. On the right side there was a cavity of large size. There was great emaciation, the pulse varied between 120 and 130, and the early morning temperature was usually about 100 and from this ran up to 103 and 103 1-2 in the evenings.

For three weeks there had been such severe dysphagia as to absolutely prohibit all eating; he had been able to drink in the Wolfenden position only.

Aphonia had been complete for seven months.

Laryngeal examination showed massive infiltration of the left ventricular band, completely hiding the corresponding vocal cord. The entire band was studded with ulcerations. Both arytenoids were edematous and covered by numerous small ulcers. The right vocal cord was ulcerated deeply along the entire edge and the interarytenoid sulcus was infiltrated and ulcerated. (Plate XIII, Fig. 43.)

Both arytenoid cartilages and the left ventricular band were thoroughly curetted and painted with pure lactic acid. Formalin, 5 per cent, was applied daily, followed by injections of orthoform emulsion, with surprising improvement as the case had been considered hopeless.

By the middle of the following month the dysphagia had disappeared, the temperature was normal and the general condition remarkably improved.

By September first he was sufficiently well to go on a long camping trip, and now after two years there is no recurrence although he has suffered several severe attacks of acute laryngitis.

CASE III.

Mrs. S., aged 29, came to Colorado in August, 1904.

There was incurable pulmonary involvement, con-**solidation and moisture to the base** on each side. with **an immense cavity on the left.**

In the larynx there was advanced infiltration with ul-**ceration of the entire edge of each** cord, ragged pro-**jections of the interarytenoid sulcus** and perichon-**dritis of the left arytenoid cartilage.**

She was given formalin rubbings followed by intra-**tracheal injections every two days.** At the end of six **months the laryngeal condition was** entirely arrested, **although the general process had grown** steadily worse. **She is still alive .and the larynx shows** no recurrence. **(Plate XIII, Fig. 44.)**

CASE IV.

E. J., a physician thirty-four years of age, was re-ferred to me in the fall of 1902.

He had had some hoarseness for several months but no pain until a few days before, when sudden and se-vere dysphagia developed. The epiglottis was swollen to several times the normal thickness, both ventricular bands were infiltrated and the left arytenoid was ede-matous. Both vocal cords were slightly ulcerated along the free edges, but there was no fulness of the sulcus, accounting for the slight disturbance of phonation.

The general condition was poor and the entire left lung was affected, with consolidation on the right ex-tending to the third rib. The usual treatment was in-stituted: daily frictions with formalin, intratracheal injections and the use at home, every three hours, of a one-half per cent formalin spray.

Within eight months there was complete arrest of the local process. (Plate XIV, Fig. 45.)

CASE V.

Mrs. R. N., aged thirty, came under observation in April, 1902. Both lungs were involved throughout, there was extreme anemia, the temperature ranged from 100 to 103 degrees, and she was obliged to do all of her housework, cooking, washing, etc.

Two-thirds of the glottis was filled by a large ragged growth that originated from and filled the entire inter-arytenoid sulcus. Both arytenoids were slightly thickened and the anterior third of the right cord, the only part of the free edge that remained uncovered, was ulcerated.

Three operations were performed upon this masss before it was entirely removed. Within four months the throat process was completely arrested and the voice normal.

She died in June, 1904, twenty-two months after the throat had been pronounced cured, and there was never any recurrence although she was forced to constantly undergo the hardest kind of household drudgery. (Plate XIV, Fig. 46.)

CASE VI.

A physician, forty-seven years of age, was first seen in June, 1904, because of a complete loss of voice that had lasted for three months.

He had had tuberculosis of the lungs for one year but there was only slight involvement at the left apex. In weight he was twenty pounds below normal.

The entire larynx, with the exception of the epiglottis, was extensively diseased. There was perichondritis of the left arytenoid, and great infiltration of the corresponding ventricular band which showed a large erosion at the most prominent point.

The right band was likewise infiltrated and ulcerated.

Both vocal cords were ulcerated at their unconcealed posterior ends and there was an ulcerated infiltrate in the sulcus.

Several extensive operations were performed, involving the partial removal of both ventricular bands, the left arytenoid cartilage and the interarytenoidal growth.

After two weeks ulceration appeared in the stump of the arytenoid, but this cicatrized later under the continued use of lactic acid and formalin.

Fifteen months after the beginning of treatment the laryngeal condition was apparently arrested, but the patient passed from observation and has not been again seen. (Plate XIV, Fig. 47.)

CASE VII.

This patient, a man thirty years of age, came to Colorado in the winter of 1902.

The laryngeal disease was so far advanced that it seemed almost useless to prescribe anything beyond cocain and morphin. At least one-third of the epiglottis was destroyed and the entire stump was covered by angry ulcers.

PLATE XIV.

Fig. 45.   Infiltration of the epiglottis and both ventricular bands, with edema of the left arytenoid. Vocal cords ulcerated and thickened.   (Case IV.)

Fig. 46.   Large warty tumor of the posterior wall; infiltration of both arytenoids, and ulceration of the anterior end of the right vocal cord.   (Case V.)

Fig. 47.   Perichondritis of the left arytenoid: infiltration and ulceration of the ventricular bands, and ulceration of the vocal cords and interarytenoid sulcus.   (Case VI.)

PLATE XIV.

Fig. 45. Infiltration of the epiglottis and both ventricular bands, with edema of the left arytenoid. Vocal cords ulcerated and thickened.

Fig. 46. Large warty t   posterior wall; infil-

anterior end of the right vocal cord.

Fig. 47. Perichondritis of the left arytenoid: infiltration and ulceration of the ventricular bands, and ulceration of the vocal cords and interarytenoid sulcus.

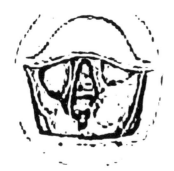

Fig. 45.

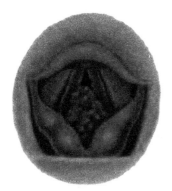

Fig. 46.

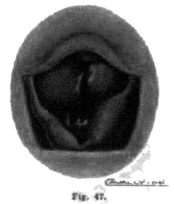

Fig. 47.

PLATE XIV.

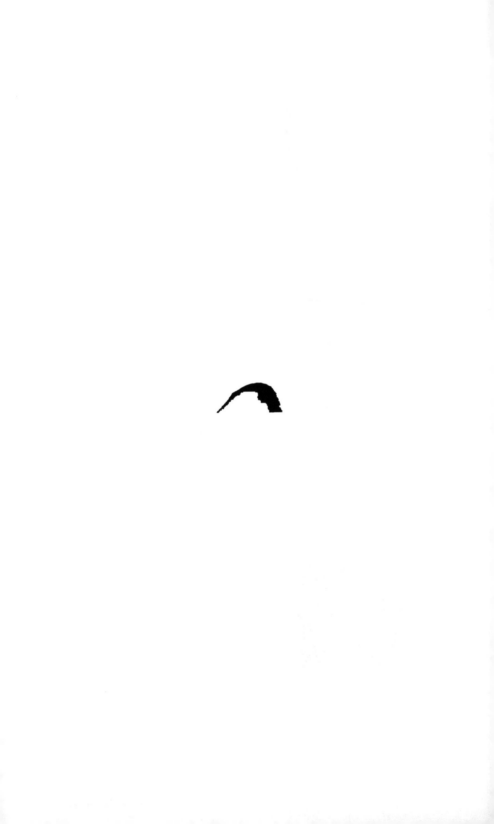

Both ventricular bands were enormously infiltrated and deeply ulcerated, completely hiding the vocal cords.

The right arytenoid was infiltrated and its entire apex was converted into a large ragged slough. The corresponding aryepiglottic fold was edematous.

The pulmonary condition was not advanced, there was only slight involvement at each apex, and the general condition was surprisingly good considering the extensive laryngeal destruction and the severe dysphagia.

The stump of the epiglottis and the right arytenoid were at once removed, the remaining ulcers were curetted and the whole larynx painted with 10 per cent formalin.

Throughout the ensuing year there was slow but steady improvement and by October, 1903, the following conditions presented: slight fullness of both ventricular bands, arytenoids normal except for a small amount of granulation tissue upon the inner surface of the right cartilage, both vocal cords ragged and thickened and the epiglottic stump entirely healed.

By March, 1904, two years from the time he first came under treatment, the laryngeal process was entirely arrested and his voice was one of unusual purity and resonance.

It remains so to this day and the pulmonary disease is likewise cured. (Plate XV, Fig. 48.)

CASE VIII.

Mrs. F., thirty years of age, had had aphonia for two years when I first saw her in December, 1903.

Both vocal cords were deeply ulcerated, giving the typical "saw tooth" appearance; the left ventricular band, which was also ulcerated, partially overhung the cord; the glottis was one-fourth filled by an ulcerated mass springing from the inter-arytenoid sulcus and the laryngeal surface of the epiglottis showed an ulcer about the size of the little finger nail.

The general condition was extremely bad: consolidation of both lungs throughout with two cavities of considerable size upon the right; high temperature and pulse, and marked anemia.

The epiglottic ulcer was lightly curetted and the formalin treatment instituted.

By the following August the left cord was entirely well and smooth, the epiglottic ulcer and those upon the left ventricular band were gone and the inter-arytenoid space showed nothing more than moderate fullness.

During all this time the general condition had grown steadily worse. When seen again, twelve months later, the larynx was in a state of arrest but it was evident that she could live but a few weeks at most. (Plate XV, Fig. 49.)

CASE IX.

H. C., a lawyer by profession, twenty-nine years of age, was referred to the author in December, 1901.

He had bilateral pulmonary involvement; had dropped in weight from 164 to 130 pounds and was a constant user of alcohol.

At the beginning of his laryngeal trouble, one year previous, there had been severe dysphagia for several weeks, but after curettement of the larynx this had

PLATE XV.

FIG. 48. Extensive destruction and ulceration of the epiglottis, massive infiltration and ulceration of the ventricular bands and right arytenoid cartilage: the corresponding aryepiglottic fold is edematous. (Case VII.)

FIG. 49. "Saw-tooth" cords: ulceration and infiltration of the left ventricular band: the sulcus is filled by an ulcerated infiltrate and there is a large, shallow ulcer on the lingual surface of the epiglottis. (Case VIII.)

FIG. 50. Infiltration of the cords, ventricular bands, sulcus and right arytenoid cartilage. The process in the cords and upon the posterior wall has advanced to ulceration. (Case IX.)

an ulcerated infiltrate and there is a large shallow ulcer on the lingual surface of the epiglottis.

FIG. 50. Infiltration of the cords, ventricular bands, sulcus and right arytenoid cartilage. The process in the cords and upon the posterior wall has advanced to ulceration.

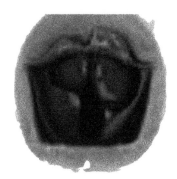

Fig. 48.

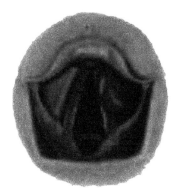

Fig. 49.

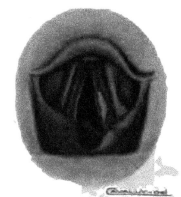

Fig. 50.

PLATE XV.

passed away and had never returned. Almost from the beginning there had been complete aphonia. Examination showed a true tuberculous ulcer in the nose, involving the anterior-inferior edge of the quadrangular cartilage and the neighboring parts of the floor of the nose.

There was ulceration and infiltration of both cords and infiltration of both ventricular bands; the right arytenoid cartilage was twice its normal size and the inter-arytenoid sulcus was filled with an ulcerated infiltrate.

The epiglottis, which I understood to be the part that had been curetted, was entirely normal.

Several months later he developed intestinal tuberculosis, but despite this the improvement in the laryngeal condition was uninterrupted and by July the throat process was arrested and the voice almost normal.

He lived until December, 1904, but there was no recurrence in the larynx. (Plate XV, Fig. 50.)

CASE X.

H. E. O'N., an electrical engineer twenty-four years of age, was referred by Dr. J. A. Wilder, in March, 1904.

There was only slight consolidation of the right upper lobe and the general nutrition was first-class.

He gave a history of having had slight hoarseness for one month and severe dysphagia for four days. The advent of pain had been preceded by a sharp chill and high fever. Before this the temperature had been normal but it now ranged from 100 degrees to 104.5 degrees.

In the larynx the following conditions were found:

Left arytenoid cartilage and the left ventricular band completely dotted with innumerable miliary tubercles; slight ulceration of the posterior ends of both cords; small mass of granulation tissue upon the inner surface of the right arytenoid; the left arytenoid and band vividly congested.

On the posterior pharyngeal wall, slightly above the tip of the epiglottis and in the median line, was a mass of similar tubercles covering an area as large as a half-dollar. Between the individual tubercles and for a considerable distance surrounding them the mucous membrane was a deep red in color and much swollen. The pain was severe and constant and the tubercles were exquisitely sensitive to touch.

By the fifth of April, thirteen days, the tubercles had disappeared, there was no pain and the temperature was again normal.

In the following September, while camping out in the mountains, he had a severe attack of ptomain poisoning and this was followed by a second crop of miliary tubercles in the larynx, but this time the pharynx was not invaded. The eruption was limited to the arytenoid cartilages.

Within a few days the tubercles over the right cartilage ulcerated, but those on the left persisted a few days longer and then gradually disappeared.

Some time later he was admitted to the Agnes Memorial Sanatorium and while there he suffered a third attack, this time with general increase of both the pulmonary and chronic laryngeal process. At the end of a year he went to Sullivan County, New York, where I

PLATE XVI.

FIG. 51. The left arytenoid and ventricular band are
vividly congested and dotted with numerous
miliary tubercules: the posterior ends of the
cords are ulcerated, and on the inner surface of
the right arytenoid there is a small mass of
granulation tissue. (Case X.)

FIG. 52. Both arytenoid cartilages are thickened, with an
extension of the edema to the right aryepiglottic
fold. Ulcerations extend over the right fold,
cartilage, cord and ventricular band. (Case XI.)

Fig. 52. Both arytenoid cartilages are thickened, with an extension of the edema to the right aryepiglottic fold. Ulcerations extend over the right fold, cartilage, cord and ventricular band.

Fig. 51.

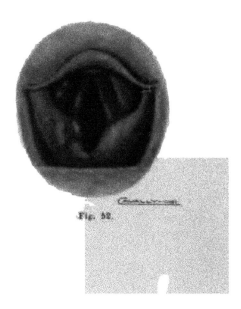

Fig. 52.

PLATE XVI.

understand he is yet living in comparatively good health. (Plate XVI, Fig. 51.)

Mrs. M., of Birmingham, Alabama, was referred by Dr. Holden, of the Agnes Memorial Sanatorium, in March, 1907.

She was suffering from excruciating dysphagia that had been steadily increasing for nearly ten weeks.

She had developed pulmonary tuberculosis over a year before, had become pregnant and was successfully delivered early in February. Three months before full term she became aphonic and developed a slight degree of dysphagia.

At the time of examination, soon after her arrival in Denver, there was complete consolidation of the right lung with consolidation and moisture of the left uper lobe. There was moderate dyspnea, extreme emaciation and depression, and the temperature rarely fell below 103 degrees. It was impossible for her to swallow anything else than thick fluids and these only with the greatest difficulty.

Both arytenoids were infiltrated and the right was the seat of three deep ulcers that covered almost the entire body. The right aryepiglottic fold was edematous and there was a small ulcer upon the right fold near the arytenoid. Both vocal cords were ulcerated and there were two small erosions upon the right ventricular band.

A bad prognosis was given and the case put under active treatment in the hope of at least partially controlling the dysphagia. Daily frictions of formalin, 3 to 10 per cent, were made, followed by the intra-tracheal injections of orthoform emulsion. A formalin spray was used every two hours and cocain given *ad libitum*. Within five weeks all of the pain had disappeared, the breathing was easy and the general condition rapidly improving.

The ulcerations of the ventricular band, arytenoid and ary-epiglottidean fold had entirely gone and the only one remaining was upon the vocal process of the left cord.

The arytenoids were still greatly thickened but the mucous membrane covering them was almost normal in color.

Regular treatment was stopped June 1st, nine weeks from the time of first examination, with the larynx in a state of virtual arrest.

Somewhat later she entered the Agnes Memorial Sanatorium, where she has remained something over three months with constant betterment of the pulmonary condition.

The laryngeal condition is still quiescent and demands no attention. (Plate XVI, Fig. 52.)

CHAPTER XI.

HYGIENIC-DIETETIC TREATMENT.

Since laryngeal phthisis is practically always dependent upon preceding pulmonary disease, no treatment can be effective unless it takes into consideration the constitutional as well as the local requirements.

Isolated cases in which spontaneous arrest result do occur, and we occasionally have the opportunity of observing a favorable issue from local treatment in an individual with whom poverty and ignorance effectually prevent the enforcement of even the basic rules of hygiene, but such exceptional cases cannot in any way invalidate the rule.

As a general proposition it may be stated that the entire result hinges upon the financial status of the individual, for all the resources of medical skill, and every climatic, hygienic and dietetic advantage must be utilized to the fullest degree. The patient should at the outset be made fully aware of the nature of the process and its gravity, for unless he appreciates the necessity for and probable duration of the new regimen, he will be unequal to the task of curtailing his pleasures and completely abandoning, for the time being, all hope of honor and emolument. That this is true of pulmonary phthisis is universally recognized and it must apply with even greater force to laryngeal tuberculosis. The chief factor in recovery is the degree of physiologic resistance inherent in the individual, and since the addition of a laryngeal focus doubles the drain, it makes essential an unusual effort towards conserving and increasing this vital force.

CLIMATE.

A suitable climate, while far from being the *sine qua non* of successful treatment, exerts a strongly beneficial influence upon the disease by reason of its remarkable power in arousing dormant energies and in stimulating metabolism. -

There has developed of late a marked and unhealthful tendency to decry the beneficial effects of selected climates and to uphold the theory of universal equality; in other words, it is maintained that it is fresh air alone and not the peculiar properties of any special atmosphere that is of value.

This question was fully considered by the Committee on Climate appointed by the National Association for the Study and Prevention of Tuberculosis, in 1905, and its report is quoted at length:

"If we look for the causes of the tendency to doubt. the value of climate they are to be found, first, in the unskillful use in the past of climate as a therapeutic measure; secondly, in the formerly widely spread belief in a mysterious specific influence of climate which led to a superstitious faith in its unaided powers and therefore to a neglect of those even more important matters, hygiene, diet, instruction and detailed supervision; third, in the effect on the general profession of their recent and all too limited experience with outdoor treatment at home, which has caused them to go from the extreme of an undue hopelessness in the past to that of an equally unwise hopefulness that any case can be cured in any atmosphere by sleeping out on a porch and eating freely.

To discuss here the various forms of climate is not within our province, but it should rather be our effort to point out what in general are the effects which in climates have a beneficial influence. These can be classified in the order of their importance, as;

First, abundance and bacteriological purity of the air; *second,* sunshine; *third,* coolness, or, in a certain number of cases, warmth; *fourth,* dryness, or, in a few cases a moderate degree of humidity; *fifth,* altitude; *sixth,* wind; *seventh,* equalibility; *eighth,* soil.

"The bacterial and chemical condition of the air has been carefully studied and has been found to vary from a very high pollution in the streets in our large cities to an almost absolute purity in high mountains, open seas, deserts, and arctic regions, and is very low in country and mountain climates, especially where sparsely settled.

"Recalling the powerful role of streptococcal and other mixed infections in pulmonary tuberculosis and their power of changing a simple tuberculosis with chronic advance into a destructive consumption, noting also the bad effects of dusty atmospheres in producing bronchial catarrh, and especially the rapid lessening of mixed infections and such catarrhs in the purer air of our mountain resorts, the importance of this factor does not need to be further dwelt upon. We would only here note that we believe it is chiefly due to reinfection of the diseased lung by pus organisms and its irritation by dust, to which is often due the relapse of some cases when they return to city life.

"After pure air we would place sunshine and sun heat, whose effects are both direct and indirect. Directly while its effects are evidently beneficial, they have never been completely analyzed and therefore will not be dwelt upon here. The indirect effects of sunshine as seen in its powerful stimulation of the patient's spirits is of great importance.

"*Dryness* in most cases is a most important factor through its valuable anti-catarrhal effects, but when extreme, this influence may be reversed and there are not a few cases in which a moderate degree of humidity is more beneficial. Generally, low humidity with moderately low temperature has a tonic effect and is beneficial in irritated conditions of the respiratory mucous membranes, while low humidity with very low temperatures, while stimulating, is apt to irritate the mucous membrane. Low relative humidity with high temperature is generally debilitating. High relative humidity with moderate temperatures are soothing to the irritated mucous membranes, but high humidity combined with low temperature favors catarrh. On the whole, in pulmonary tuberculosis, low relative humidity with moderately low, or low, temperature is most generally suitable and the average tubercular patient always makes his best gains in cold, dry weather, where such conditions prevail, but there are certain cases who do better with a high relative humidity and warm temperature.

"*Equalibility* in older people or in the very feeble

can be of great value, but is not as important as used to be supposed. In stronger cases variations in temperature stimulate the vital activities, hence, generally speaking, equalibility is not an important factor.

"*Wind,* when the patient is directly subjected to it, is harmful, but when he is properly protected its purifying influence on the air, provided vegetation is sufficient to prevent dust storms, is beneficial.

"*Altitude.* Most authorities are agreed that other things being equal some degree of altitude owing to the great purity of the air and to its stimulating effect on the metabolism and appetite, etc., is most desirable, but it is not here our function to discuss the large question that this opens up. Enough to say that care should be used to choose an altitude to suit the patient's degree of vitality and heart-power."

This report has been quoted in full because it points out the necessity of climatic treatment in all curable cases of pulmonary tuberculosis, and because as a general proposition it may be advanced that the climatic conditions best suited for the pulmonary disease are most helpful for the concomitant laryngeal lesions, and as it has been proven that every pulmonary patient financially able should seek a new and more favorable climate from that in which the disease developed, it is therefore manifest that all cases of laryngeal tuberculosis, not hopelessly incurable, should be sent to that locality best suited to the pulmonary and general condition.

Above all else, the termination of a laryngeal lesion is dependent upon the progress of the general disease, hence any measures advisable in the latter condition are suitable for the throat. A few exceptions are to be noted: .

A continuous out of door life despite the conditions of the weather is advisable in practically all cases of pulmonary tuberculosis and is, therefore, generally indicated in laryngeal cases, but where there are advanced and painful lesions, the patient is more comfortable in a perfectly lighted and ventilated room unless the weather is moderate and equable.

If the lesions are acute and the larynx highly inflamed, the atmosphere should be kept moist and fairly warm.

No matter how advanced the condition, unless there is acute inflammation, the patient must be kept constantly in the open air except during periods of high winds, dust storms, extreme cold, and sudden variations in temperature.

Contrary to the generally accepted theory that laryngeal patients do best in a moist, warm climate, it has been the author's experience that the exact opposite is true, especially with the still curable cases.

In the late stages of the disease, when widespread ulcerations exist, the moist warm climates of the Southern coasts are more soothing than the dry and stimulating air of the uplands, but in such instances it is a question of euthanasia and not of cure. As long as there is the slightest prospect of either permanent or even temporary arrest, the patient should seek that locality most suitable for the pulmonary disease without considering the larynx itself, except that he should not be sent beyond the reach of skilled laryngological supervision, or into those arid sections where the humidity is extremely low and where, because of lack of vegetation, dust storms are of frequent occurrence.

A strongly unfavorable prejudice exists regarding the influence of high altitudes upon laryngeal tuberculosis but it can be easily demonstrated that this is entirely unwarranted; we have only briefly to consider the percentage of arrested cases in the so-called favored climes, in comparison with those reported from all other sections, to show that the higher altitudes not only render arrest or cure more probable but that they also confer a certain degree of immunity.

Observers resident in the high altitudes report an approximate percentage of 60 in permanent arrests, as against an average of 15 per cent from all other sections of the world.

These more favorable results cannot be ascribed to a possibly average milder type of the disease or to a greater proportion of incipient cases, for the exact opposite is liable to obtain because of the fact that these favored areas have long been dumping grounds for the indigent consumptives of the entire country.

Levy (N. Y. Med. Journal, Nov. 1, 1902) from a large series of cases, arrived at the following conclusions:

1. "In cases in which both the lung and throat lesions develop in Colorado, the throat lesion manifests itself 48 weeks later than in those originating elsewhere."

2. "In cases in which the lung lesions develop elsewhere and the throat lesions in Colorado, the throat lesion manifests itself 62.3 weeks later than in those originating elsewhere."

The author's cases give approximately the same results. On the other hand, such authorities as Lake and Schech strongly advise against high altitudes, and the latter recommends a moist, dust free atmosphere, and particularly long sea voyages.

Low humidity with moderately low temperature is best in the majority of throat cases, and as with the lungs, the greater degree of improvement is usually made during the cooler months.

The conditions in Denver, where the larger part of the statistics employed in the chapter on Prognosis were gathered, can be seen from the following reports of the United States Weather Bureau. The average of the two years, 1904 and 1905, has been taken:

MONTHLY SUNSHINE.

	July	Aug.	Sept.	Oct.	Nov.	Dec.
Per cent.	65.	64.	70.	74.	76.	68.

	Jan.	Feb.	Mar.	April	May	June
Per cent.	58.	64.5	45.5	53.	60.	67.5

MONTHLY A. M. AND P. M. HUMIDITY.

	July	Aug.	Sept.	Oct.	Nov.	Dec.
6 a. m., degree	72.	69.5	65.5	72.	61.	59.5
6 p. m., degree	41.5	41.	36.5	47.5	40.5	49.

	Jan.	Feb.	Mar.	April	May	June
6 a. m., degree	68.	68.	80.5	69.	74.5	69.
6 p. m., degree	53.	45.	57.5	48.	44.5	37.5

MONTHLY PRECIPITATION.

	July	Aug.	Sept.	Oct.	Nov.	Dec.
Inches	1.84	0.63	1.13	1.35	0.04	0.20

	Jan.	Feb.	Mar.	April	May	June
Inches	0.58	0.20	2.47	4.31	2.05	2.06

MONTHLY WIND MOVEMENT.

	July	Aug.	Sept.	Oct.	Nov.	Dec.
Miles	5254	5079	5172	5431	5426	5813

	Jan.	Feb.	Mar.	April	May	June
Miles	5452	5196	5598	5564	5439	5476

The author has had several opportunities of studying these cases during periods of residence in comparatively high altitudes, 6000 to 8000 feet, and never was there an appreciably unfavorable influence exerted upon the larynx, except in patients with advanced and incurable lesions of an ulcerative type. In these instances the dry and cold air caused some irritation and increased pain, as was proven by their partial amelioration upon going to sea level.

This experience has been the same throughout the mountains of Colorado, New Mexico and Arizona, except in those localities where vegetation is very sparse, for in such places the almost constant presence of dust in the atmosphere caused considerable irritation. The warm, moist air of Southern California seemed to exert a singularly soothing influence upon cases with advanced ulceration.

The open air treatment in any climate, if rigorously enforced, has a marked deterent effect upon the development of laryngeal tuberculosis.

In commenting upon the statistics gathered from thirteen British sanatoria relative to the development of laryngeal phthisis during the open air treatment, Lake (Laryngeal Phthisis, Pg. 52) says:

"From this table it will be seen that out of 1,979 patients, who neither had laryngeal infection at the time of admission, nor were attacked within two weeks from that time, only 22 became infected during the ensuing four months, a proportion of 1 in 90."

While it has been impossible to get definite statistics from many of our American sanatoria, it is the almost unanimous opinion that tuberculous infection of the larynx rarely occurs in patients who have carefully adhered to the out-of-door, rest regimen for a number of weeks.

Whether the patient remains in the place where the disease was contracted or seeks a new climate, he should at the outset spend some months in a well conducted sanatorium. In no other way can he learn so readily and thoroughly the proper mode of living; knowing the correct rules is not usually sufficient, the habit must be firmly fixed.

Particularly is this true in connection with complete vocal rest, as few patients will submit voluntarily to this necessary regulation, and hopeful results are not to be anticipated unless absolute and prolonged abstinence from speaking be enforced.

DIET.

The diet should conform to that indicated in pulmonary phthisis but when dysphagia supervenes certain modifications become essential.

Owing to the mechanical hindrance to deglutition and the resultant nasal regurgitation, and to the pronounced aversion to eating consequent upon the severe pain attending every effort at swallowing, both the quality and quantity of the food, as well as the method of taking it, demand careful regulation.

The bulk must be reduced to a minimum while the nutritive value is maintained by the highest possible concentration, at the same time keeping the food bland and unirritating. It must not be too hot nor too cold; too thin nor too solid; too sweet nor too sour, and all spices must be omitted. Nothing that acts as a mechanical, thermic or chemical irritant should be used.

Thus the problem of how to supply the proper nutritive values and at the same time tempt the appetite by a variety is exceedingly difficult, and only possible in the milder degrees of dysphagia.

Thin liquids occasion more trouble than the more solid foods, hence substances of a semi-solid or thick fluid nature must be the main reliance.

First of all and the basis of nearly all these foods, is milk: If the digestion is unimpaired it is best given in the form of cream, and preferably, in so far as the throat is concerned, in large doses at long intervals rather than in the ordinary manner of small amounts frequently repeated.

This naturally puts a severe strain upon the digestive organs, but sipping is practically out of the question as in nearly all these cases fluids must be taken in large gulps.

Various preparations of milk or cream whereby the consistency is increased and a variety offered, are available. Thus koumiss, junket, egg nog, and dry bread soaked in milk and squeezed dry before eating, are of occasional service. The following recipes have been used with good effect:

NUTRITIOUS COFFEE.

Dissolve a little isinglass in water, then put one-half ounce of freshly ground coffee into a sauce pan with one pint of new milk, which should be nearly boiling before the coffee is added. Boil for three minutes, clear, add the isinglass and allow it to settle. Beat up an egg and pour the coffee mixture upon it.

CREAM LEMONADE.

Beat up the white of one egg, add three teaspoonfuls of sugar and the juice of one lemon. Pour over one-half glass of cracked ice and add four ounces of cream.

MILK PORRIDGE.

Tie some flour in a bag and boil from four to five hours. Grate to a powder and mix into a smooth paste with cold water. To four ounces of milk add one pint of water and stir in the flour. Boil ten minutes, constantly stirring.

A preparation that has been found to be both nutritious and easily swallowed can be made according to the following formula:

Mix 2 heaping tablespoonfuls of Eskay's or some similar food with one-half pint of cool water and make a smooth, thin mixture; then boil in a double boiler for forty minutes, cool, and add two eggs, previously well beaten, and mix. If desirable, add a tablespoonful of Angelica, Tokay or Muscatel Wine.

Nothing is swallowed with greater ease than oils, hence the preparation of Olive Oil and eggs, under the name of Egmol, prepared by Park, Davis & Co., is valuable.

Nutritious soups and bouillons can be given the proper consistency by the addition of sago, tapioca, oat meal or gumbo. They should be served moderately cool and without pepper.

Custards, jellies, and either wine or coffee gelatin, are grateful and may be easily swallowed by those with only moderate involvement. Even in the severest cases meat in the form of "Biftick a la Tartare" can occasionally be eaten.

Two ounces of raw meat from which all the gristle and tendons have been removed, is finely minced and thoroughly mixed with the yolk of an egg. This is eaten cold, without seasoning, either alone or spread upon thin slices of buttered bread.

Beef juice can be given at intervals.

Calves' brains, butter, kefir and calves' foot jelly are likewise palatable and are eaten with comparative ease.

Malt extract is nearly always well born and is sometimes more easily swallowed than milk.

In advanced cases of laryngitis thirst is always a distressing symptom because of the attendant pyrexia, copious, tenacious secretions and the small amount of liquids taken. The thinner the fluid the harder it is to swallow, hence water cannot be taken in satisfying quantities. Luke warm or cold coffee, chocolate and almond milk are agreeable substitutes and are more easily taken than water.

Acid drinks would be indicated were it not for the severe pain they produce, but this effect is partially counteracted by their mixture with cream or milk in such a way as to avoid curdling. The cream lemonade is one of the best of these preparations; the recipe for another follows:

WHITE OF EGG LEMONADE.

Take two lemons, the whites of two eggs, one pint of boiling water and sugar to taste. The lemons must be peeled twice, the yellow rind being utilized, while the white layer is thrown away. Place the sliced lemon and the yellow peal in a jug with two lumps of sugar, pour the boiling water on them and stir occasionally. When cooled to about the ordinary temperature of tea, strain off the lemons. When the lemonade is in full agitation by whipping, add slowly the white of egg and continue whipping for two or three minutes. While

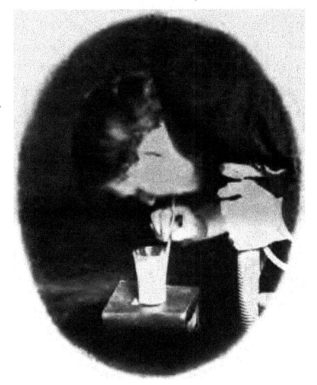

Fig. 53.

still warm, strain through muslin. Serve when cold.

Small ice pellets slowly dissolved in the mouth afford temporary relief.

Ice used in this way for half an hour before eating, or in the form of compresses about the throat, will slightly lessen the pain on swallowing.

METHODS OF EATING.

As before mentioned, fluids can be swallowed much more easily by "gulping" than by sipping.

If regurgitation or severe pain can be avoided in no other way, the patient should lie prone upon a sofa with the head well beyond the edge and somewhat be-

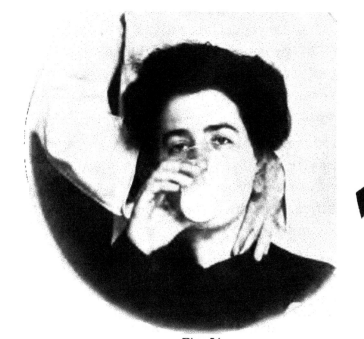

Fig. 54.

low the level of the body, and suck the fluid through a long glass tube. (Fig. 53.)

While this is often of service it fails in the majority of cases.

Deep pressure exerted upon the sides of the neck by the palms of the hands, pressing inward and forward from behind. and lifting the larynx away from the pharynx, often assists deglution to a slight extent. (Fig. 54.)

When all other methods have failed life may be prolonged by feeding through the stomach tube and by nutritive enemata. The former method is usually inadvisable in that it is distinctly repugnant to most patients, the passage of the tube is painful and it cannot prolong life more than a short time at most. There can be but two possible indications: temporary feeding after laryngeal operations and the occasional necessity of prolonging life to the utmost, but the practice of forcing nutrition in this way, when no hope of even temporary improvement is held, is generally reprehensible.

When the necessity of prolonging life does arise, as well as in the first few days succeeding radical operative procedures, nutritive enemata will meet all the requirements and occasion much less discomfort and repugnance.

Any of the following standard preparations can be used:

1.—Eggs, two to three; 20 per cent grape sugar, one-half cup; Red wine, one glass; starch, a thimbleful.—Ewald.
2.—Milk, 250 grams; egg yolks. two; salt, a pinch; Red wine, dessertspoonful; starch, dessertspoonful.—Boas.
3.—Milk, 250 grams; starch, 60 to 70 grams.—Leube.
4.—Milk, 250 grams; Peptone, 60 grams.—

5. Crush one pound of beef, add one pint of cold water and allow to macerate three-quarters of an hour. Raise to the boiling point and boil two minutes. Give four ounces every four hours. Use tepid.

TOBACCO AND ALCOHOL.

All cases of laryngeal tuberculosis are better off without tobacco in any form, but if the amount of involvement is slight and the patient long addicted to its use, moderate smoking can do no particular harm, especially if a thoroughly cleansed pipe with a long stem be used in the open air.

After the use of tobacco in any form the mouth and throat should be well washed with a mild antiseptic solution.

If for any reason alcohol is indicated it should be given in the mildest forms and well diluted with water.

The harmful effects of excessive indulgence in spirits are as pronounced upon the laryngeal lesions as upon the constitutional malady and should be absolutely prohibited as a regular habit.

VOICE REST.

The influence of complete vocal rest upon the course of the disease is not generally appreciated and cannot be exaggerated. If the lesions are incipient and not progressive, moderate use of the voice may be permitted, but all singing, reading aloud and prolonged conversations must be strictly enjoined.

If, on the other hand, the process is moderately advanced and active, absolute rest is imperative if the best results are to be attained.

All conversation should be carried on by writing and the finger manual, or in some cases by whispering. In the latter case the whisper must be soft and low, for a loud or forced whisper is as harmful as ordinary speech.

Even in the incipient stages arrest will be more certain and prompt if absolute prohibition of speaking is enforced, and it is perhaps no exaggeration to say that this is the *one* most valuable agent in the management of these cases.

NASAL AND PHARYNGEAL HYGIENE.

In all cases of laryngeal tuberculosis the mucosa of the entire upper respiratory tract must be kept in as nearly a perfect condition as possible.

Mouth breathing, permanent or intermittent, nasal suppuration, or naso-pharyngeal and pharyngeal catarrh naturally exert an unfavorable influence upon both the laryngeal and general condition, and should therefore be corrected unless there is some potent contra-indication. The mere presence of a tuberculous lesion in the larynx does not make inadvisable the surgical correction of obstructive and suppurative conditions of the nose or pharynx, providing the general nutrition is good, the temperature not high, and that there is no organic involvement other than the pulmonary. If the laryngitis is acute the correction of such morbid processes should be postponed for the time being, and any surgical interference is inadvisable in cases of far advanced disease, but in all cases where arrest of the laryngitis is possible the establishment of normal respiration is imperative.

If an operation is indicated it should be the simplest consistent with thoroughness, even if the subsequent condition is not made ideal.

The object is not to make an anatomically perfect nose but a physiologically good one, and in the great majority of instances this can be accomplished by measures so simple as to cause little discomfort and drain upon the patient's strength.

Thus, if occlusion is due to a moderately deflected septum, such operations as the submucous resection and those requiring the wearing of tubes for considerable periods, should give way to compensatory turbinectomies, the removal of spurs, etc.

Hypertrophied tonsils, lingual glands, etc., must likewise be removed if they are accountable for any marked local or reflex trouble.

Enlargement of the lingual glands is especially liable to aggravate the laryngeal disease, because of the fact that in the vast majority of instances in which the glands are sufficiently enlarged to touch the free edge of the epiglottis, they provoke an almost incessant cough that is of itself enough to cause considerable irritation and congestion in the larynx.

These glands are enlarged to some extent in almost all cases of tuberculosis, although not sufficiently, as a rule, to cause epiglottic pressure, and are themselves frequently the site of tuberculous changes.

Showing the frequency of this involvement we have the statistics collected by Freudenthal. He says, "At the City Home, where we have only advanced cases, 33 patients were examined and only eight were found negative, i. e., without an enlarged tonsil. The other 25 had all marked hypertrophies of the tonsillar tissues of that region.

"At the Bedford Sanatorium 86 patients were examined (males and females), of which 59 were in the so-called first stage of pulmonary tuberculosis, 20 in the second stage, 5 in the third, and 2 unclassified. Of these 63 were found to have a markedly enlarged lingual tonsil, while of the rest—(23)—the majority showed some hypertrophy, those having normal conditions being the exceptions.''

In fifteen consumptives examined by Dmochowski, the lingual glands were tuberculous in nine.

In conclusion we can sum up by saying that the entire upper respiratory tract must be put into the best possible condition for the same reason that the normal functions of all organs must be maintained, if the general tuberculous process is to be conquered.

CHAPTER XII.

MEDICINAL TREATMENT.

The medicinal treatment is naturally considered under two heads: constitutional and local.

1. Constitutional.

It is not within the province of this work to consider the various so-called "specifics," suffice it to say that as yet none of these agents has shown an appreciably curative influence upon the larynx.

Krause (Berliner Klin. Wochenschr., No. 42, 1902) claims to have observed a favorable action in tuberculous laryngitis from the intravenous injection of sodium cinnamate, or hetol. Practically all other observers, however, have had negative results, and in the few cases that have come under my observation no reaction whatever has been observable.

Several experimenters, notably Pottenger, of California, have reported enthusiastically upon the favorable effects of tuberculin, and Von Ruck's watery extract. Pottenger says:

"The preparation that I have used for the most part is the watery Extract of Tubercle Bacilli (Von Ruck's). The larynx is the ideal location for a lesion to be treated by tuberculin for the dosage can be controlled absolutely by the local reaction produced

The larynx should be watched daily, and the dosage should not be increased beyond that which is necessary to produce a slight local reaction; nor should a second injection be given until all reaction produced by the first has disappeared.

"Tuberculin administered in this manner will cure many cases of tuberculous laryngitis. It will increase the chances of recovery from fifty to seventy-five per cent, and in many cases it will offer practically the only hope."

Von Ruck himself claims remarkable curative powers for his preparation. Before the National Association for the Prevention of Tuberculosis, he said:

"As regards the treatment of these cases (laryngeal) the great majority require no local measures whatever. Immunization with the watery extract is all that is essential, except in instances in which the disease has advanced to the stage of massive infiltration and deep ulceration. In such cases palliative measures to relieve the distressing symptoms are of course indicated."

On several occasions the author has selected a considerable number of these cases, typifying each stage of the disease, and has had them treated by tuberculin, keeping the larynx under daily observation. In not a single instance was there any notable improvement, at least in excess of that which usually occurs in patients who are placed under the best of hygienic conditions, but without treatment other than enforced vocal rest, cleansing sprays, etc., and these measures were enforced in every case.

The great majority of laryngologists have experienced similar negative results, and for this reason tuberculin is seldom used at the present time except for diagnostic purposes.

As with all innovations, the treatment by bacterial vaccines, controlled by the opsonic index, is now being eulogized as a specific in laryngeal as well as in pulmonary phthisis, but as yet we have no statistics that justify the claim and we are not warranted, at the present time, in considering the treatment as anything more than an adjuvant that may be of occasional service.

General medication, with the view of exerting any direct effect upon the larynx, is useless, excepting in so far as two indications are to be met, i. e., the control of cough and the facilitation and lessening of expectoration.

Both of these objects are important, for the difficulty of causing cicatrization in a broken down tissue subject to incessant irritation by coughing and the passage of tenacious and infectious secretions is easily appreciated, and while this applies especially to lesions that are advanced and painful, it is also applicable to those of an incipient character.

For the cough either heroin or codein should be given in doses sufficient to reduce it to a minimum.

Lozenges containing menthol, orthoform, etc., are sometimes of considerable service in allaying cough due to laryngeal or pharyngeal irritation.

When expectoration is excessive the internal use of creosote or guaiacol, preferably in the form of the carbonates, creosotal and duotal, is indicated. The former, in doses of five drops after meals, gradually

increased to thirty drops, and the latter in doses of
0.2 to 0.5, three times daily, increased to 1 to 2 gm.,
sometimes have a marked effect in reducing the quantity of sputum, and in allaying cough.

To facilitate expectoration hot drinks are especially
useful. A spoonful of whiskey in a glass of hot milk,
or ten to thirty drops of aromatic spirits of ammonia,
with a pinch of salt and soda bicarbonate in a glass
of hot water, may be used for this purpose.

The choice of local treatment depends upon the
extent of the pulmonary process, upon the vigor of
the individual, and upon the extent, character and
location of the laryngeal lesions.

It would manifestly be irrational to apply the
same principles of treatment to the patient with advanced pulmonary disease, high fever, emaciation,
etc., as to one with an incipient lesion, high vitality
and normal temperature. In the former instance
the aim is euthanasia if the patient is absolutely
doomed, or palliation and curative treatment sufficient merely to hold the local lesions temporarily stationary if there is yet some hope of arresting the lung
disease; in the latter case vigorous and sustained
curative treatment is indicated.

The remedies are applied in the following ways:

(1.) Inhalations.
(2.) Sprays.
(3.) Insufflations.
(4.) Pigments.
(5.) Intratracheal injections.
(6.) Submucous injections.

Before considering these different methods in detail, the fact should be emphasized that no drug, no matter how employed, has any specific action upon the disease and that therefore none of the appended agents can be considered directly curative in any sense; they act by maintaining asepsis to a certain degree, by relieving pain and cough, by stimulating sluggish ulcers and by promoting absorption and fibrosis, and within these bounds only may they be looked upon as curative.

So many "cures" have been proposed, so many agents recommended, that no serviceable purpose can be fulfilled by giving them all in detail, therefore only those substances will be considered which have proven of some service in the author's practice.

INHALATIONS.

Steam inhalations are of considerable use in allaying an associated catarrh, in cleansing erosions and in favoring expectoration. To a slight degree they promote temporary anesthesia. For the latter purpose the most active drug is anesthesin, which may be used in one of the following mixtures:

```
Anesthesini............................. 5 drs.
Mentholi................................ 3 drs.
Ol. Oliv. .............................. 4 fl. ozs.
```
Or

```
Anesthesini............................ 45 grs.
Sp. vini. rect. ....................... 1½ fl. ozs.
Aq. destil. ........................... 2 fl. ozs.
```

Inhale for ten minutes.

Either of these preparations will produce a very slight degree of anesthesia, sometimes lasting as long as two or three hours. Orthoform may be substituted for the anesthesin in either of the mixtures.

The inhalation of any one or more of the essential oils; pine, eucalyptus, peppermint, sandalwood, etc., or of Comp. Tincture of Benzoin, assists to some extent in combatting the accompanying catarrhal conditions. After the use of any vapor the patient must remain indoors for at least a half hour, and the inhalations may be repeated as often as every two to five hours.

SPRAYS.

The chief advantage of the spray correctly used is the possibility, through its instrumentality, of keeping the larynx free of mucus and pus, an absolute essential of successful treatment.

To maintain cleanliness it must be used every two to four hours and considerable practice is required before the solution can be made to thoroughly bathe the entire larynx. Any non-irritant antiseptic may be used, my preference being for formalin, two to three drops to the ounce of the following detergent solution:

```
Sodii biboratis.
Sodii bicarbonatis ........................ aa gr. x
Acidi carbolici ........................... gtt. iii
Glycerini ................................. 3ii
Aquae destil. q. s. ad. fl................. 3i
```

Following the cleansing solution a camphor-menthol spray in oil is of some service.

In dysphagia, to keep the pain in subjection and to make deglutition possible, the spray is invaluable. Cocain, 1 to 5 per cent, according to the degree of involvement, is the mainstay, but its unpleasant after effects of dryness and seeming constriction often render its use inadvisable.

Alypin, 1 to 10 per cent, is a valuable substitute; its anesthetic properties are only slightly inferior to those of cocain, and while the taste is equally unpleasant it is only in the exceptional case that it causes constitutional depression.

The action of all the anesthetics is enhanced by occasional change from one to the other.

INSUFFLATIONS.

The insufflation of various powders is one of the oldest, and most ineffectual, of the methods of introducing medicaments. By "auto-insufflation" it is possible for the patient to draw a considerable amount of powder into the larynx. One end of a straight glass tube some six inches long is pushed into the powder until a sufficient amount is forced into the bore, the opposite end is then passed well back into the mouth, the lips and nose are tightly closed, and a deep inspiration taken.

The powder is drawn into the larynx and is retained for a considerable period, often many hours.

Iodoform, the powder most universally used, is irritating, frequently produces a troublesome cough and is destructive to the appetite, so should rarely be employed.

Orthoform and anesthesin, thoroughly dusted upon the ulcerated mucosa, produce some relief of pain, much more evanescent, however, in the author's experience, than is commonly reported. A lasting anesthesia of from eighteen to thirty-six hours is said to be frequent, but according to my observations, three to four hours is an uncommonly long effect, and even during this short period the relief afforded is insignificant. In many cases they are entirely ineffectual.

None of the powders affect intact membranes and as they are mostly non-poisonous they can be used in any quantities and as frequently as desired. The continued use of orthoform, however, seems to have a slight disintegrating effect upon the ulcers and should not be used over long periods.

Morphin is not generally satisfactory because of its constitutional effects and unfavorable influence upon the pulmonary secretions.

Thiocol, highly praised by Fasano (*Arch. Internae. di Med. et Chir., XVI., Napoli,* 1900) has not seemed to do any particular good, and the same may be said of the various iodine compounds; iodol, aristol, and traumatol; of resorcin; chinosol, a quinin derivative, and of amyloform, a combination of formaldehyde and starch.

Almost the sole sphere of the insufflation seems to be in the home use of the anesthetic powders, and even for this purpose their use should be greatly restricted, as the soothing inhalations and anesthetic sprays are more effective and do not produce the irritative cough that so often follows the introduction of dry powders.

PIGMENTS.

In so far as medicinal treatment is concerned, the one really effective procedure is the direct application of the various pigments. Both the methods of using and the drugs to be employed demand careful consideration.

After witnessing the manner of making applications in vogue with a large number of laryngologists, particularly in tuberculous cases, the conclusion is irresistible that faulty technique is responsible for such a large percentage of innocuous effects.

Even at the present time it is next to impossible to purchase an applicator that is of the slightest use in treating laryngeal lesions of a tuberculous nature. The ideal instrument must combine sufficient strength to permit of firm pressure and "scrubbing," with

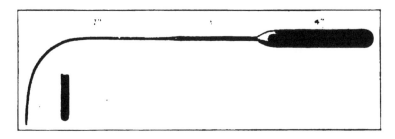

Fig. 55.

enough elasticity to prevent the possibility of making surface abrasions; it must at the same time be light in weight and large enough to handle with a firm grasp. (Fig. 55.)

Those purchasable at the instrument dealer's are either of thin flexible wire of little resistance and strength, or of hard and rigid steel that cracks and breaks after slight use.

With an instrument of proper size and flexibility, applications can be made with sufficient firmness to force the pigment well into the tissues, a *sine qua non* of successful treatment.

As well try to heal an old syphilitic ulcer of the leg by applying ointments without preliminary preparation of the surface, as to affect a sluggish tuberculous ulcer or infiltrate by too gentle manipulation, yet almost all writers on tuberculosis warn against "active interference" with the lesions, be they acute or chronic.

In the majority of instances applications should be made at frequent intervals employing solutions of moderate strength, rather than at longer periods with more powerful ones.

Except when it is desirable to produce a strongly caustic action daily frictions are generally advisable. The object is to maintain a continuous effect without promoting undue reaction; if this occurs complete rest must be given for some days.

It often requires a considerable nicety of judgment to determine the point beyond which reaction must not be allowed to progress. When we are dealing with a case of angry ulcerations attended with swelling and severe subjective manifestations, an increase in both the subjective and objective symptoms due to over zealous manipulation might easily be considered simple progression of the tuberculous condition and lead to even more active interference.

The following case well illustrates this point:

"Mr. P., salesman, thirty-four years of age, came under treatment for a moderately advanced tuberculous laryngitis. Both vocal cords were infiltrated and ulcerated along their free borders, there was considerable swelling of the interarytenoid sulcus, and both ventricular bands were irregularly ulcerated and moderately thickened. For six weeks he was treated daily by vigorous applications of 5 to 10 per cent formalin, with constant increase in the subjective symptoms. Each seeming advance brought an increase in the vigor with which the treatment was pursued.

"Upon the development of alarming dyspnea, tracheotomy was advised and the case referred to me for operation. The larynx was closed, except for a pin-point opening, by the angry ventricular bands, which were covered with minute ulcerations. The vocal cords were completely hidden and the arytenoids were edematous and deeply ulcerated. Operation was deferred, antiphlogistic treatment instituted, and in ten days the dysphagia and dyspnea had completely disappeared. The condition upon the subsidence of these acute symptoms corresponded largely with that recorded at the primary examination, except that the ulcerations were slightly deeper and more extensive. Within six months after the renewal of the old treatment, upon a somewhat less vigorous scale, the larynx argyrol and nargol, phenol, para-mono-chlor-phenol, no recurrence."

The pigments most commonly used are lactic acid, formalin, ichthyol, resorcin, guaiacol, pyoktanin, argyrol and nargol, phenol, para-mono-chlor-phenol and Iodine Vasogen.

LACTIC ACID.

Since the year 1885, when Krause (*Milksaure g. Larynxtubercul. D. Med. Woch.*) advanced the claims of lactic acid as a curative agent, and demonstrated upon the cadaver the presence of healed tuberculous lesions where the acid had been used during life, it has held first place in treatment. In lesions of an ulcerative type it has but one equal, formalin, but unlike the latter it is valueless in cases with intact epithelium.

In sensitive patients the primary application should be with a solution of not over 20 per cent strength, although a preparation as weak as this has but slight curative value.

The concentration should be rapidly increased to the full pharmacopeial strength. Considerable misapprehension exists as to the required frequency of applications, it being used in many instances as often as three times a week.

Lactic acid exerts a cauterizing effect upon an abraded surface with the formation of a thin scab which, as a rule, is not thrown off for about seven or eight days and sometimes not until as late as the second or third week. Beneath this scab, in favorable cases, healthy granulations form and new epithelium extends from the edges of the ulcer with final transformation into scar tissue. Until the scab has separated additional applications are valueless.

The pain attendant upon applications of lactic acid is due to the ulcerated areas for it has no effect upon normal tissue, hence these spots should be well anesthetized, both in order to prevent suffering and to permit careful manipulation under guidance of the mirror. In no other way can the application be effectively made.

To act upon a non-ulcerative area the lesion must

first be converted into an open wound by scarification, as was the practice some years ago, or the diluted acid must be thrown into the tissues by means of a syringe and needle. The introduction of more penetrating agents has rendered both of these procedures unnecessary, although the latter method is still used to some extent.

FORMALIN.

Since the year 1897, formaldehyde has almost entirely supplanted lactic acid in the author's practice, both in the ulcerative and infiltrative types, with ever increasing satisfaction.

While in no way a specific it is the nearest to the ideal of any drug we possess, in that it is effective in every type of lesion in a degree equal, if not superior to, any other agent. Upon ulcers it is as effective as lactic acid used in corresponding frequency and concentration, and possesses the marked advantage of causing comparatively little reaction and no pain of any moment. It is, therefore, possible and advisable to apply it daily, or at the least thrice weekly, in a strength varying from 3 to 10 per cent.

In a number of almost parallel cases, one-half treated with lactic acid and one-half with formalin, as well as in a considerable number of individuals treated alternately with the two drugs, the formalin almost invariably gave the better and more prompt results.

A typical case from these records, demonstrated by the author at the 1904 meeting of the American Academy of Ophthalmology and Oto-Laryngology, is quoted from the *Laryngoscope*, of October, 1904:

"Mr. W. M., jeweler, 32 years of age. In January, 1902, six months after pulmonary tuberculosis was diagnosed, there developed complete aphonia with considerable dysphagia and two months later, upon his arrival in Denver, he presented the following picture:

"Entire epiglottis deeply ulcerated with loss of nearly one-half its substance; ventricular bands so infiltrated as to partially overlap the cords, with ulceration at the most prominent point of each. The left arytenoid twice the normal in size and extensively ulcerated. Both cords infiltrated and ulcerated throughout with considerable masses of granulation tissue at their posterior attachments. The interarytenoid sulcus infiltrated and ulcerated.

"Treatment, of which formalin constituted the most important part, was instituted with considerable improvement at the end of three months. At this time lactic acid was substituted, with the occasional use of guaiacol, with continued retrogression, when at the end of eight weeks the use of formalin was resumed. By the following January the ulcerations were healed except for one small spot on the under surface of the epiglottis, while the infiltration of the ventricular bands had almost disappeared.

"At this time I left the city for four months and the patient was under the care of an experienced colleague, who having no faith in this treatment used lactic acid and methylene blue. Upon my return the throat was worse than at the first examination and a hopeless prognosis was again made. Under the old treatment, however, the condition rapidly improved, and six months later he accepted a position as a salesman in a large jewelry store which he has since uninterruptedly held.

"In examining the larynx to-day, were it not for the distorted epiglottis and slight scarring at several points, one could have no suspicion that it had ever been the seat of tuberculosis."

Formalin, in a strength of from 3 to 5 per cent, can be used daily, thus maintaining a continuous influence, an effect impossible of attainment with lactic acid, and to this continued action, I believe, can be credited much of its really remarkable power.

In lesions of an infiltrative and vegetative type formalin is more generally effective than any other pigment, although in certain cases one of the other drugs may be more useful.

When vegetations and infiltrations are localized or excessive they should be surgically removed, providing the general conditions are favorable, but after all the tissue capable of surgical treatment has been dealt with, or primarily in case operative procedures are contra indicated, the frequent use of formalin is generally advisable.

This favorable action is likewise shown by its effect upon aural granulations, whether tuberculous or simple inflammatory.

The continued use of formalin is said to favor the development of dry gangrene, a result never seen by the author nor by any of his immediate colleagues. As a prophylactic agent it is unexcelled and its constant use in a one-half per cent solution, in the patient's hands, will save many a suspicious case from infection and many an incipient one from further development.

It is strongly antiseptic in weak solutions. In a strength of 1 to 10,000 it prevents the development of bacteria and it is germicidal in a 1 to 75,000 solution.

A 1 to 10,000 solution arrests the growth of the germs of anthrax, cholera, typhoid, and the staphylococcus pyogenes aureus.

Its advantages may be summed up as follows:

(1) It surpasses all other bactericides in solutions of a strength which can be tolerated.

(2) In tuberculous ulcers it is fully the equal of, and probably superior to lactic acid.

(3) Its effect upon vegetations is prompt and pronounced.

(4) In infiltrative cases it is by far the most satisfactory remedy.

(5) It is the only drug of the curative class that can with safety be placed in the hands of the patient, thus making it possible to maintain a continuous cleansing, germicidal and absorbent action.

(6) Its field of usefulness comprises all the varied types of the disease.

The formalin solutions should be freshly made every two or three days, and the applications of the stronger solutions should be preceded by cocain, as they occasion sharp pain for several minutes, both laryngeal and aural.

ICHTHYOL AND RESORCIN.

Ichthyol and Resorcin, 10 to 20 per cent, have been used to a considerable degree in non-ulcerative lesions of moderate extent, with fairly satisfactory results.

GUAIACOL AND CREOSOTE.

Guaiacol and Creosote, recommended especially by Chappell, Vacher, and Sendziak, are used in strengths ranging from 1 to 10 per cent. In the author's hands they have not proven satisfactory.

PYOKTANIN.

Pyoktanin, used upon ulcers, either in concentrated solutions or fused upon wire, is sometimes beneficial, although greatly inferior to lactic acid, formalin, and the phenol compounds. It can be used as an antiseptic spray in 1 per cent solution, and has been strongly endorsed by Sheinmann, Schech (*Handbuch Der Laryngologie*, 1898) and Rosenberg (*Behandl. d. Kehlkopftubercul. Ther. Monatsch.* 7-9, 1888.).

NARGOL, ARGYROL AND PROTARGOL.

These organic silver salts, 1 to 20 per cent, are of considerable service in the so-called "pre-tuberculous stage," that is, where there is chronic congestion and relaxation of the mucous membranes without definite tuberculous changes. They exert no appreciable influence when ulcerations have developed, nor in cases with marked tumefaction.

PARA-MONO-CHLOR-PHENOL.

Para-mono-chlor-phenol is of use in both the ulcerative and infiltrative lesions. It is caustic in action when used as strong as 10 to 20 per cent. Simanowski (*Ueb. d. Behandl. Phthisis u. anderer Erkrank. d. ob. Luftwege, m. Ortho-u. Para Chlor Phenol. Centralbl.*

f. Lar. XI, 1895) prefers it to all other caustics and it
is also well recommended by Hedderich, Seifert, Zinn,
Spengler and Richards.

IODINE-VASOGEN.

Iodine-Vasogen, a 10 per cent preparation of iodine
dissolved in vasogen, is of some service in cases of
beginning infiltration, and in painful swellings about
the arytenoidal joints. The vasogen is more penetrating than the other media and the preparation is entirely painless.

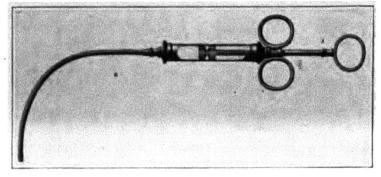

Fig. 56.

Of all these remedies, those that have proven most
effective in the author's practice and stand out pre-
eminent, are formalin, lactic acid, ichthyol and iodine-
vasogen.

INTRATRACHEAL INJECTIONS.

One of the most satisfactory methods of introducing
medicaments into the larynx and trachea is by means
of the intratracheal syringe. (Fig. 56.)

Originally introduced for the cure of pulmonary
tuberculosis, it has to-day taken its rightful place as an

invaluable addition to the armamentarium of the laryngologist.

Under direct illumination the point of the syringe is carried well down between the vocal cords and the injection is made while the patient takes a deep inspiration. The solutions, in considerable quantities, penetrate into the larger tubes and minute amounts reach the remote alveoli. There is rarely any spasm, at least in excess of that occasionally produced by the simple laryngeal spray.

As a rule the cough is markedly decreased, and the sputum is lessened in quantity and becomes less tenacious; the oily covering of the larynx protects it to a considerable extent against the irritant secretions, and the sensation of tickling in the throat and suprasternal notch is often removed for many hours.

The treatment is both curative and palliative. If topical applications are made at the same sitting the injection should be given last.

Any of the following solutions may be used:

```
1.—Menthol.................................. 30 gr.
   Guaiacol................................. 10 gr.
   Ol. Sassafras............................
   Ol. Cubebs.............................. aa gtt. iii
   Glymol.................................. 1 oz.

2.—Camphor-menthol........................ x to 60 grs.
   Olive Oil .............................. 1 oz.

3.—Guaiacol............................... 9 parts
   Eucalyptol ............................. 2 parts
   Menthol ................................ 1 part
   Saturated sol. of Iodoform in ether to.....100 parts

4.—Olei thymi, Olei eucalypti, Olei cinnamonii. aa gtt. lxxx
   Iodoform................................ 15 grs.
   Olei olivae steril. .................... ℥ iii
```

Both of the following preparations are especially valuable in dysphagic cases.

```
5.—Menthol.................................... *1 part
    Almond oil  ............................. 30 parts
    Yolk of egg  ............................. 25 parts
    Orthoform  .............................. 12 parts
    Water to.....................................†100 parts

6.—Menthol.................................... 1 dr.
    Anesthesin............................... 5 drs.
    Ol. oil.................................... 4 fl. ozs.
        *Increasing to 15 parts.
        †Freudenthal.
```

All of the solutions should be used warm, between 80 and 90 degrees F., and from ¼ to 1 ounce can be injected at a sitting.

When successfully made a feeling of warmth extends through the entire chest and when any of the pungent drugs are used they are frequently tasted, after coughing, from twelve to twenty-four hours. A second injection may be given as soon as the good effects of the preceding one have worn off, daily, or even twice daily if possible.

SUBMUCOUS INJECTIONS.

The use of sub-mucous injections for the cure of non-ulcerative infiltrations of the larynx was introduced by George Major in 1886 (*The Treatment of Laryngeal Tuberculosis by Submucous Injections of Lactic Acid, Canadian Med. and Surg. Journal*, Dec. 1886).

In the following year the method was indorsed by both Heryng and Krause. In this country Chappell has been the leading advocate, and in England, Watson Williams.

A special syringe (Fig. 57.) is used and a few drops of the selected solution are thrown into the tissues at those points where the submucous tissue is most abundant. The needle is introduced about one-half centimeter and the injections are made at intervals of not less than eight to ten days.

The different experimenters have used different agents; Major, Heryng, Krause and Gleitsmann use from 3 to 5 drops of a 10 per cent solution of lactic acid; Watson Williams, guaiacol, or 2 per cent aristol in almond oil, or perchloride of mercury, 1 in 1,000 of glycerine and water; Störk employed a sublimate solution; Lake a 20 grain to the ounce solution of chloride of zinc, and Chappell, 1 to 4 minims of creosote

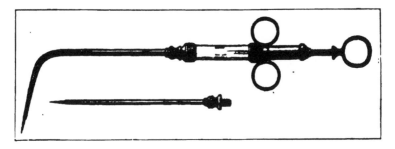

Fig. 57.

or guaiacol in oil. Solly (*Laryngoscope,* June, 1904) advised the use of 20 minims of a 15 per cent solution of lactic acid.

The following formula has been employed by Chappell:

```
Creosoti  ................................. ʒi-ii
Ol. gaultheriae  .......................... ʒiii
Ol. ricini  ............................... ʒiii
Paraffini liquidi  ........................ ʒi
Menthol  .................................. x grs.
```

All of these substances when injected into the tissues produce severe pain and inflammation, with the formation in many cases, of large superficial sloughs. Because of this they should always be used in localities rich in submucous tissue.

The results are rarely satisfactory, the reaction is too severe and better methods are available, hence the treatment has fallen into some disrepute and is not used as freely as a decade ago. The author has used lactic acid and guaiacol to some extent, but sometime since abandoned both as highly unsatisfactory.

The daily use of the penetrating pigments, especially formalin, supplemented by the frequent spraying with the formalin-detergent solution, has been much more effective than the submucous injections, is painless, and has no harmful consequences. In case of extreme infiltration the removal of tissue by the cutting forceps is by far the preferable procedure.

PHOTO-RADIO-THERAPY.

Ever since Roentgen's discovery of the X-ray, continued efforts have been made to cure laryngeal tuberculosis by this and other rays with, it cannot be denied, only indifferent results.

A voluminous literature has accumulated, a perusal of which forces the belief that while certain rays may in some cases favorably influence pain, cough and expectoration, they exert little or no visible effect upon the diseased tissues.

The Finsen light, high frequency current, Minin light, search light, sun light and radium have all been used to a certain extent.

THE X-RAY.

In the author's experience the Roentgen rays have proven almost invariably disappointing. When employed upon incipient lesions no effect whatever has been observable, while in the advanced cases, those associated with ulceration and marked infiltration or edema, the reaction has often been sufficient to provoke new activity with increase in both the subjective and objective symptoms. Unless carried to the point where some reaction was observable, no apparent influence was exerted.

The majority of experimenters have had similar experiences and as a result its use has been largely abandoned by laryngologists, even by those who were in the beginning most enthusiastic.

Pancoast (*Phila. Med. Society,* April 26, 1905) reported one case of at least temporary cure. This patient had ulceration of the epiglottis and a tuberculoma of the anterior commissure, with consolidation and softening of the right apex.

Applications of the X-ray, of five minutes' duration, using a medium vacuum tube having a resistance of about 3 inches of spark gap, with the anode placed 12 inches from the patient, were made during a period of seven months. At this time the pulmonary lesion could scarcely be located and Dr. Harland reported the larynx cured. Pancoast also reports several additional cases in which marked retrograde metamorphosis occurred.

The rays to be effective must be used externally, for Roentgen himself showed that they cannot be polarized, deflected nor concentrated by lenses, hence it is not possible to deflect them into the larynx by means of a laryngeal mirror.

The Finsen light and Minin light have even less influence than the X-rays and therefore do not demand separate consideration.

RADIUM.

Theoretically, radium should be the most practical radio-active substance for use in laryngeal phthisis, in that the rays can be brought into direct contact with the diseased tissues; they travel in straight lines and cannot be deflected except by a magnet. It is too early as yet, however, to draw definite conclusions concerning its efficacy, although in the few cases to which it has been applied the results were negative.

J. C. Beck (*Trans. Amer. Academy Ophth. and Oto-. Laryng.* 1904) reported one case of laryngeal tuberculosis with dysphagia in which radium alone failed to give any relief, but combined with other treatment seemed more effective than when local medical treatment alone was used.

In a case of primary tuberculosis of the nasal septum, accompanied by severe pain in the frontal region and some difficulty in breathing, he applied the radium 33 times, in the beginning every day, then three times a week and finally once a week. He says:

"The headaches and pain disappeared after the second treatment. After about six treatments the mass looked better and did not bleed as easily on touch. After twelve treatments the patient was able to breathe better, but far from free, and from this time on, until three weeks ago, which terminated the thirty-third treatment, the improvement as to diminution in size of the growth has not been perceptible. The appearance of the mass was improved. It appeared harder and looked as though the mucous membrane was going to cover it. Later treatment by the X-ray failed to induce further improvement."

The technique is simple: 50 milligrams of radium of the 10,000 radio-activity, placed in a tube, is brought into contact with the diseased tissues and allowed to remain from five to thirty minutes.

SUNLIGHT AND ARC LIGHT.

The searchlight and the direct or reflected sun rays have been used with occasional good effect in so far as the relief of pain and some lessening of cough are concerned.

Freudenthal, who has had a wide experience with the electric light, summarized his views (*New York Med. Journal*, July 12, 1902) as follows:

"I can see in the electric light only an adjuvant that is of great assistance in the management of some cases of tuberculosis."

During a period of nearly two years the author used the concentrated electric light rays in a large number of cases and finally abandoned the treatment as practically valueless. That it had a favorable influence upon pain cannot be denied, and occasionally the cough was somewhat lessened and expectoration favored, but aside from these effects it seemed to be entirely without action and it has been possible to obtain these results in higher degree by other and much less fatiguing treatment.

The sunlight treatment has been highly recommended by Sorgo of the Alland Sanatorium, who claims to have seen essential improvement in all of 14 cases so treated. His patients sit with their backs to the sun and the light is reflected into the larynx from a mirror mounted on a stand. With a laryngoscope in position, the patient controls the reflection of the rays by the image he obtains of the larynx. Sorgo says:

"The results have surpassed all expectations. Essential improvement was obtained in every case. The best results were apparent in tumor-like infiltration of the laryngeal mucosa, while diffuse red infiltrations of the vocal cords yielded more slowly. The difference between the response of these two forms was most marked when both co-existed in the throat. The specific action of the sunlight was particularly apparent in two cases in which the patients, from lack of skill, failed to expose more than a certain part of the vocal cords. The exposed area showed marked improvement, while a sharp line divided the improved, exposed area from the unexposed unimproved part.

"The moral effect of this sunlight treatment on the patients is good. They see the infiltration subsiding, and, although the voice may still be hoarse, yet they know they are improving. They soon acquired the knack of this autolaryngoscopy. The number of exposures ranged from 6 to 44, during from two to six months."

Autolaryngoscopy, to the extent of a patient directing his own treatment and noting the improvement therefrom, does not appeal to the experienced laryngologist as a practical procedure and hence one is not inclined to give much weight to these statistics.

When the sunlight treatment first gained prominence and was almost universally employed, both in the form of direct rays and by reflection from large concave violet mirrors, the author saw a considerable number of laryngeal patients who were receiving daily exposures of from thirty minutes to two hours. In not a single instance was there the slightest change in the appearance of the involved tissues; in several there was some lessening of dysphagia but not to as great an extent as was later observed from applications of the concentrated rays of the arc light.

CHAPTER XIII.

SURGICAL TREATMENT.

ENDOLARYNGEAL OPERATIONS.

Since the year 1880, when Moritz Schmidt first advocated the employment of deep incisions for painful swellings of the epiglottis and posterior wall, the question of surgical intervention in tuberculous laryngitis has been subject to endless controversy, with the decision, in so far as the great majority of laryngologists is concerned, still in abeyance.

The ultra enthusiastic hopes engendered by the communications of Krause and Heryng have not been fulfilled, but on the other hand, the extreme pessimism incident to the non-realization of these early anticipations has given way to a moderate optimism, based upon the accumulated experiences of twenty years.

The indications and contraindications for operative interference are of infinitely greater importance than the method of operating itself. In deciding upon the advisability of surgical intervention two indications must be kept constantly in view; the relief of pain, and the cure or temporary arrest of the disease.

If the former indication alone is to be met, no consideration whatever need be paid to the general condition of the patient aside from his ability to withstand the shock of the operation. We are confronted by a single problem and that concerns the probable degree of relief to be anticipated.

It may be definitely stated that in general radical extirpation or division of the involved tissues will produce more or less complete relief of dysphagia, more lasting and effective than it is possible to obtain from any other system of treatment.

Medicinal treatment is generally ineffectual in the severer cases of dysphagia and accomplishes little beyond momentary control, and in consequence, any procedure that offers promise of even partial relief must be considered a boon and this we undoubtedly possess in some one or more of the various radical operations. Even though the requisite operations shortened life they would still be indicated, but in practice they are found to prolong it and remarkable cures occasionally result even in apparently hopeless cases.

If cure or arrest of the local disease is still probable, a number of conditions must be taken into consideration unless the surgical interference is to consist of nothing more than simple curettage of sluggish ulcers, indolent granulations, or small and sharply circumscribed infiltrations.

The following rules are generally applicable:

(1) The lesions must be surgically incipient, that is, they must be accessible and fairly well circumscribed.

Only a localized lesion can be thoroughly eradicated and complete removal is advisable although not invariably essential. It is not always possible to judge accurately of the boundaries of a seemingly localized lesion, for the infiltration usually extends much farther than is evidenced by the laryngeal image, and an approximately correct estimate is possible only to one with considerable clinical and pathological experience.

Widespread infiltrations and ulcerations associated with high temperature and dyspnea are absolute contraindications, but the rule cannot be held as applying to those advanced cases that have resisted all other treatment.

(2) The lesion must be accessible.

Occasional barriers to thorough endolaryngeal curettement are found in such conditions as a narrow and distorted larynx; a rigid or laterally compressed epiglottis; an unfavorable location of the lesion, and excessive reflex irritability, uncontrollable by cocain, where every effort at manipulation is provocative of violent attacks of retching and coughing.

(3) The pulmonary process must be either incipient or quiescent.

The condition of the lungs merits even more consideration than the extent and character of the local lesion itself. Advanced pulmonary disease or a less extensive condition that is rapidly progressive usually renders surgical work of any kind inadvisable but the statement made in connection with the surgically incipient lesions may be here repeated; none of these indications and contraindications can be held as valid when the lesions have already proven resistant to other treatment, or when they are the cause of severe and otherwise unconquerable pain.

(4) Extensive operations should not be performed upon one with organic tuberculosis other than pulmonary.

(5) Those patients who show a marked reaction to cocain, i. e., cardiac weakness, fever, insomnia and loss of appetite, must not be subjected to secondary operations unless some one of the newer and presumably non-poisonous anesthetics proves effective and harmless. These cases are very rare but of considerable importance, for when cocain, or the operation itself, plays havoc with the nervous and digestive systems, it is foolhardy to persist in its use, for the loss in general vigor will more than outweigh any possible local improvement.

The entire subject may be condensed by saying that no radical procedures for the cure of the larynx should be undertaken that entail heavy expense upon the part of the lungs or the general strength; it avails nothing to cure the larynx and at the same time cause permanent progression of the general disease.

In an individual, however, who meets all the above requirements, early and complete removal of all diseased tissue is always indicated provided a fair trial of simpler treatment has been unavailingly made.

The choice of operation depends upon the preferences of the individual operator, and upon the size, location and character of the lesion but as a general rule, it may be claimed that the use of cutting instruments in far preferable to electric cauterization or electrolysis. These may supplement but should rarely supplant the methods that aim at thorough removal rather than the slow destruction of the diseased tissues, for complete extirpation should be the objective no matter how extensive the measures demanded.

The reaction from galvano cauterization is fully as great as from the cutting operations and a dozen applications will not as a rule accomplish more than one fearless removal of tissue. Electric or chemical cauterization, however, should generally succeed the radical operations, in order to destroy any tissue that may have escaped the knife.

OPERATIONS.

The operations are classified as endolaryngeal and extralaryngeal.

The endolaryngeal operations are:

(1) Incision and scarification.
(2) Curettage.
(3) Galvano cauterization.
(4) Electrolysis.

The extralaryngeal operations are:

(1) Tracheotomy.
(2) Intubation.
(3) Thyrotomy.
(4) Laryngectomy.

INCISION AND SCARIFICATION.

Simple deep incisions have an extremely limited field of usefulness. Even Moritz Schmidt, who introduced the treatment for the relief of dysphagia dependent upon edematous infiltrations of the epiglottis, aryteno-epiglottidean folds and posterior wall, has abandoned it to a large extent.

As a pure palliative procedure it has some merit in a limited type of cases; those in which dysphagia depends upon extensive infiltration of the posterior wall. With a pair of angular scissors an incision is made through the laryngo-pharyngeal wall, down to and including the interarytenoid incisure.

Under 20 per cent cocain anesthesia the pain is not severe and usually completely disappears by the end of the second or third day. For from three days to a week feeding by the rectum is necessary, by which time the edges of the wound will have united firmly enough to permit the swallowing of liquid and semi-solid food.

The relief of pain is generally marked, temporary arrest of the process is not extremely rare and instances of enduring cure are on record. Hemorrhage and the falling forward into the larynx of one flap are the only accidents to be apprehended. Bleeding is never uncontrollable and the forward displacement of a flap can usually be avoided by maintaining a recumbent posture during the period of healing; if this fails the prolapsed part should be removed with the double curette.

Deep incisions have sometimes been advantageously employed in cases of smooth diffuse infiltrations as a preliminary to the use of lactic acid, but since the introduction of the more penetrating pigments the method has become largely obsolete.

In edema scarification causes considerable shrinkage with a corresponding decrease of the subjective symptoms. Either a single deep linear incision or multiple punctures can be made.

A deep incision into the epiglottis extending from free edge to base will oftimes relieve the dysphagia due to tense infiltrations or perichondritis, but it should only be made when for any reason complete amputation seems inadvisable.

CURETTEMENT.

The term curettement embraces excision as well as simple scraping or evidement.

Of all endolaryngeal surgical procedures it is the one most commonly employed and most generally useful. Introduced to the profession by Heryng in 1887 (*D. Heilbark. d. Larynx Phthisie*), it has steadily gained wider acceptance until its general worth is now almost universally acknowledged, although it must be admitted that in America surgical treatment has not gained the recognition accorded it on the Continent.

Local anesthesia is a necessary precursor of every laryngeal operation and must be sufficiently complete to destroy all mobility and reflex irritability. For the more delicate maneuvers the pharynx and palate must be included in the anesthesia. The larynx is first sprayed with a weak solution of cocain or alypin, 2 per cent, until superficial sensibility is deadened, then repeatedly mopped with a 10 to 20 per cent solution.

The simultaneous use of adrenalin chloride, 1 to 10,000, increases the effectiveness of the cocain and permits of the operation being concluded without the field becoming obscured by blood. At the same time it decreases the chances of constitutional depression.

In exceptional cases, even when a 20 per cent cocain solution has been freely used, the mere introduction of an instrument will produce an immediate cramp of the glottis; in such cases the cocain will have to be introduced by submucous injection.

The hypodermic administration of morphin and atropin, thirty minutes before the operation, is particularly serviceable in nervous patients and in those in whom it is desirable to prevent a free excretion of mucus.

A full half hour is commonly required before the larynx can be brought under perfect control. Constitutional effects are rare, much more so, in fact, than from the use of corresponding amounts in the nose and pharynx.

Preliminary cleansing of the larynx, except for the removal of mucus and pus at the time of operation, is unnecessary. The use of creosote and iodoform for five or six days preceding operation, as advised by Mascarel (*Traite chirurg. d. végetations d. l. laryngite tubercl. Thèse* Paris, 1890) and Castex (*Traite chir. d. l. phthisie lar. Ann. d. mal de l'or,* July, 1893), is purely gratuitous, as a single act of coughing immediately before or during the operation renders the larynx as septic as if preliminary cleansing had been entirely omitted.

INSTRUMENTS.

The instruments required include single curettes, double curettes or cutting forceps, knives, and galvanocautery points and snare. The two sets of curettes known as the Heryng and the Heryng-Krause meet all requirements and are universally applicable.

The former consists of knives and single curettes of various sizes and shapes, attachable to a universal handle and adjustable at any desired angle. (Fig. 58.)

The Heryng-Krause instruments, comprising the double curettes or tube forceps, may likewise be at-

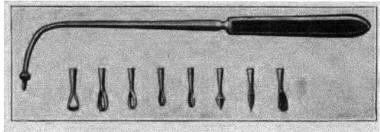

Fig. 58.

tached in any position to a universal handle. (Fig. 59.)

The set of double curettes made by Pfau are admirably suited for the more delicate operations. (Fig. 60.)

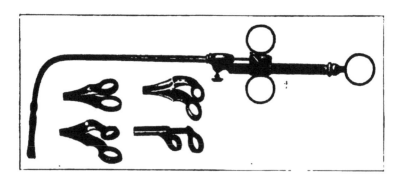

Fig. 59.

To replace the tube forceps Lake has designed various punch forceps which are of considerably greater power.

The first of these has an oval cutting edge set at an oblique angle with the shaft and is designed for operations upon the interarytenoidal region. (Fig. 61.)

Fig. 62 shows a powerful forceps of large size for excision of the epiglottis.

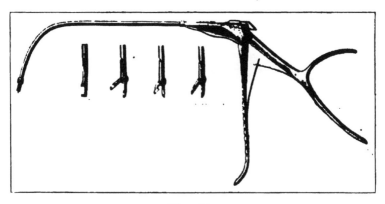

Fig. 60.

The third instrument (Fig. 63) has a circular cutting edge and is designed for any part of the larynx above the rima glottidis with the exception of the interarytenoid sulcus.

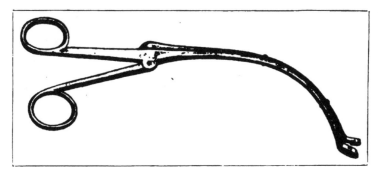

Fig. 61.

For removal of the epiglottis either the forceps or the galvano-cautery snare (the Schech handle is most convenient) can be used.

The author has modified the familiar lingual tonsillitome to fit the epiglottis and has found it more gener-

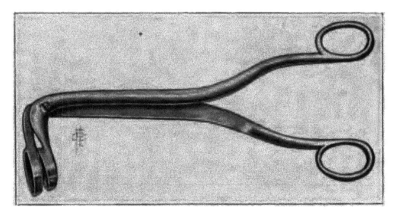

Fig. 62.

ally satisfactory than any of the punch forceps. It removes nearly all of the organ in one piece, the detached part cannot fall into the larynx, and the operation is

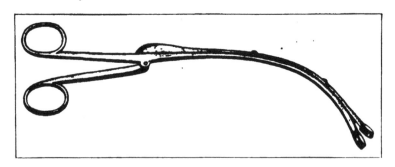

Fig. 63.

performed with great rapidity and a minimum of pain, desiderata of great value in most cases. (Fig. 64.)

INDICATIONS FOR SIMPLE CURETTEMENT.

(1) Removal of friable granulations and tumors.

(2) Removal of sharply circumscribed infiltrations.

(3)   Stimulation and cleansing of sluggish ulcers.

Curettement, when thoroughly done, is sometimes a procedure of considerable difficulty. The tuberculous larynx is often exceedingly sensitive, so irritable in fact, that despite thorough cocainization, every effort at manipulation provokes uncontrollable seizures of coughing and cramp.

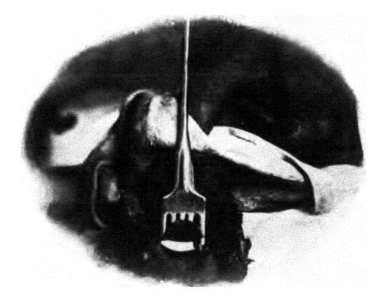

Fig. 64.

This is especially true of lesions involving the posterior wall and interarytenoid - incisure, success, in some instances, following only after repeated attempts. Many skilled laryngologists support this view, notably Schech (*Handbuch der Laryngologie, Pg.* 1168), Krieg (*Ueb. Ort. Behandl. d. Kehlkopf. tuberc. Corr. Bl. f. Wurtz. Aerzte, Nr.* 32, 1894) and Hajek (*D. loc. Behandl. d. Kehlkopf. tuberc. Centralb. f. ges. Ther. Nr.* 2, 1895).

Schäffer (*Ueb. d. Curettement d. Larynx. Ther. Monatsh.*, Oct., 1890) admits that it is generally easier for him to remove a laryngeal polypus, no matter where situated, than to properly curette a tuberculous lesion that extends well down in the interarytenoid sulcus. This point has been particularly emphasized because curettement is usually looked upon as the simplest of laryngeal operations, to be performed by every novice in laryngology.

The consistency of the growth must always be taken into consideration, for with the single curette it is practically impossible to remove some infiltrates, i. e., those tough, firm swellings of the posterior wall that bear a strong resemblance to true fibrous or scar tissue. Neither can it be satisfactorily employed upon the free edge of the epiglottis nor upon the tip of the arytenoid cartilages, owing to their non-resistance to firm pressure.

The lesions most adapted to simple curettement are localized infiltrations and sluggish ulcers of the true and false cords, the laryngeal surface of the epiglottis, and the interarytenoid sulcus. Acute lesions, those associated with edema and high fever, generally contraindicate currettage.

Thoroughness is an absolute essential and a second scraping is permissible, if necessary, as soon as the slight reaction consequent upon the preceding operation has subsided. Immediately after the operation, pure lactic acid or 10 per cent formalin should be thoroughly rubbed into the wound.

EXCISION.

Excision is the method *par excellence* in those cases in which complete removal of the morbid tissue is possible.

Contrary to the usually accepted dictum that excision should be limited to those cases with sharply circumscribed lesions, the author frequently operates, with good effect, upon patients in whom the disease is so extensive as to preclude the possibility of complete extirpation.

This is only done, however, when all other treatment has proven ineffectual, or in cases with obstinate dysphagia. Partial removal, except in cases with extremely numerous and disseminated foci, renders the remaining tissue more amenable to medicinal treatment.

That this procedure is sound has been repeatedly demonstrated in the author's practice. It must be admitted that this is directly contrary to the experience of almost all laryngologists and these more favorable results must undoubtedly be due in large part to climatic influences.

Many objections have been raised to any radical operative interference:

(1) The danger of causing increased activity in the pulmonary disease or of producing general tuberculosis.

(2) The impossibility of removing all diseased tissue.

(3) The proven fact that recurrences are frequent.

(4) The technical skill requisite for operating.

(5) The danger of infecting new tissue.

(6) That the mere removal of tuberculous tissue does nothing to prevent new infections from the lungs.

In regard to the first and most valid objection little of real value can be adduced. In a few cases there has been a post operative exacerbation of the general process, but such careful observers as Heryng, Gleitsmann and Krieg, hold that a connection between the two has not been proven and that the increase in pulmonary activity might well have been accidental.

On the other hand, Rethi, Lermoyez and Sokolowski have seen cases in which the dependence of the general infection upon surgical procedures seems to have been definitely established.

In a large series of operative cases the author has never met with one, where the general nutrition was fairly good and the lung condition quiescent, in which any harmful effects from the laryngeal work became evident. In a number of cases of advanced pulmonary disease the operations did unquestionably cause some temporary activity. While the danger is a possible one, it is extremely remote and should never be allowed to interfere with a necessary operation; laryngeal tuberculosis, of itself, often leads to excrutiating pain and death unless vigorously combatted and checked, and hence a slight possibility of disseminating the infection cannot be considered a valid contra-indication.

Schrötter based his objections to surgery upon the assumption that the tuberculous tissue cannot be so thoroughly removed as to eliminate all possibility of recurrence. It is true that recurrences after one to five years are distressingly frequent, but it is equally true that the percentage of enduring cures is not increased by other methods of treatment, and in the majority of instances in which the disease has reappeared, it can be shown that life has undoubtedly been prolonged, and much suffering averted, by reason of this early intervention. Moreover, many cases have been completely cured that would have otherwise succumbed.

Neither is a complete extirpation essential to temporary arrest or even to absolute cure. Most gratifying results are sometimes attained in patients where a partial removal of diseased tissue is followed by long periods of medicinal treatment and the author, personally, no longer seriously considers the extent of involvement, provided it is not so widespread as to absolutely preclude the possibility of benefit.

When there is generalized extrinsic, or combined extrinsic and intrinsic infection, it is self evident that endolaryngeal surgery should be limited to those procedures requisite to the relief of dysphagia, but one should not be invariably deterred by the simple fact that a lesion has progressed beyond a point permitting of complete removal.

Excision of a ventricular band, of an arytenoid cartilage or an ary-epiglottic fold can rarely be complete, yet their partial removal, even when extensively diseased, results frequently in complete healing or, at the least, prepares the way for more successful medicinal treatment.

Partial removal is advisable in all cases of even extensive involvement provided medicinal treatment and simple curettement have failed, for chemical agents then become more effective and the patient is not alone given a better chance of complete or temporary arrest but of more prompt relief as well.

Immediate cure is not to be thought of in any case, prolonged after treatment being an invariable essential no matter how thorough the excision.

That an operation demands unusual skill upon the part of the surgeon cannot be held as a rational argument against its performance, for few of the life saving operations can be performed with equal skill by all surgeons, and each must necessarily be left to those especially equipped by nature and training.

That there is danger of infecting new tissues is theoretically correct but its occurrence in practice has rarely been observed, and the same holds true in regard to the liability of causing mixed infection.

In extralaryngeal operations infection of the line of incision is not rare and offers one of the strongest objections to such methods but in endolaryngeal work it is extremely uncommon even when preventive measures have been neglected. The wound, even when much diseased tissue is left, heals promptly as a rule.

Some twenty-four amputations of the epiglottis have been made by the author without in a single instance having an infected stump, and practically every case was complicated by advanced pulmonary disease and involvement of other segments of the larynx.

The chief danger lies in wounding the epiglottis, either through prolonged pressure or direct traumatism, but this can usually be avoided by correct and careful technique.

To the last objection, i. e., that the removal of the tuberculous tissue does not prevent new infections from the lungs (Solly, Laryngoscope, June, 1904) it need only be said that the same objection applies with equal force to all other treatments.

Should all intervention be therefore abandoned?

The indications for the use of the double curette, as given by Schech, are:

(1). Removal of circumscribed or not too diffuse infiltrations of the epiglottis, ventricular bands, the posterior wall and ary-epiglottic folds.

(2). Ulcerations of the epiglottis, aryepiglottic folds and arytenoid cartilages accompanied by severe dysphagia.

(3). All cases of infiltrations and granulations which because of their consistency cannot be removed by the single curette.

As already mentioned, ulcerations or limited infiltrations of the tips of the arytenoids and the edge of the epiglottis, cannot be satisfactorily removed with the single curette; with the double instrument, however, the required amount of tissue can be easily excised.

Complete amputation is nearly always indicated when there is extensive involvement of the epiglottis. In such cases, because the rest of the larynx has usually already succumbed, the prognosis is highly unfavorable and little can be expected from operative treatment aside from the relief of pain. A not inconsiderable number, however, approximately 10 per cent, are permanently cured, a much better showing than that made by other methods of treatment.

The cures are naturally most liable to occur with those in whom the remaining segments of the larynx are not extensively involved. The results are usually

AFTER TREATMENT.

The larynx must be given complete rest for several days.

Immediately succeeding the operation, pure lactic acid or formalin, 10 per cent, should be applied thoroughly, followed by the insufflation of orthoform and aristol. The larynx is also to be sprayed at intervals of two to three hours with an alkaline solution containing one-half per cent of formalin.

If there is marked inflammatory reaction, adrenalin chloride, 1-10,000, used as a spray at frequent intervals, is of decided benefit, and inhalations or injections of menthol in oil are temporarily soothing.

The local application of cocain and morphin is sometimes necessary, and rectal feeding is advisable for two or three days, although not invariably essential.

The reaction, however, is usually slight and constitutional symptoms, i. e., headache, fever and prostration, exceptional.

The temperature occasionally rises from one to three degrees, but persists for not more than one or two days.

Hemorrhage is rare and when it occurs is easily controlled. Heryng has seen but two severe cases in 270 operations, both occurring after removal of the ventricular bands. Moritz Schmidt has also had but two cases.

If severe bleeding does occur adrenalin chloride should be freely applied, and if this proves inoperative, equal parts of lactic acid and sesqui chloride of iron.

GALVANO-CAUTERIZATION.

Galvano cauterization has an important though extremely limited field of usefulness. The lesions to which it is particularly adapted are dense firm infiltrations of the ventricular bands, anterior commissure of the cords, and subglottic region. It is also of occasional service in promoting cicatrization of unduly sluggish ulcers, although for this purpose the curette is more generally applicable and effective.

The cutting away of the ventricular bands is liable to provoke considerable bleeding, hence in these cases the use of the cutting forceps has in large part been superseded by electric cauterization. In the subglottic region and at the anterior commissure it is largely a question of accessibility; if the infiltrated tissues cannot be grasped by the forceps they must be destroyed, in so far as possible, by the cautery.

For dysphagia dependent upon infiltration of the posterior wall, both Gleitsmann and Price-Brown advocate the use of the cautery, a procedure which the author cannot unequivocally endorse. In such cases, if the infiltrate is sufficiently massive to require numerous deep punctures, the reaction may be so severe as to materially increase the dysphagia for some days, and the results are generally less satisfactory than from the more radical procedures. The cauterization may be made with complete safety, however, when the lesions are only of moderate extent, and in such cases may be of considerable service in helping to differentiate between the thickenings due to early tuberculosis and chronic catarrhal laryngitis.

In applying the cautery the point must be buried deeply in the tissues, penetrating as nearly as possible to the base of the lesions, the number of punctures depending upon the extent of involvement. Edema rarely occurs, there is no danger of after infection, and the pain is not severe.

Secondary applications are not allowable until after complete separation of the resultant scab.

ELECTROLYSIS.

Although the destruction of tuberculous tissue by electrolysis has been advocaed since the year 1889, the method has never become popular owing to the uncertainty of the results, the time consumed in treatment, and the pain inflicted.

It possesses no advantages over the true surgical precedures, except in rare instances, and in these the indications are more effectively, and more promptly met, by galvano-cauterization, i. e., firm infiltrations that cannot be grasped by the forceps, and in localities where incision is likely to provoke hemorrhage.

Simple infiltrations of the vocal cords that resist medicinal treatment occasionally respond to electrolysis, but even in these cases cauterization is more effective.

Opinions as to its usefulness are not unanimous, however.

Kafemann (Ueb. Electrolyse. u. i. Anwend, b. Erkrank, d. Nase u. Rachens m. spec. Berücks, d. Lar. tubercul. Ther. Monatsh. 1893) formerly recommended electrolysis for hard, tumor-like infiltrations of the ventricular bands, for chorditis vocalis inferior, for tumor-

like swellings of the aryepiglottic folds, and for flat
infiltrations of the epiglottis. His early favorable im-
pressions, however, were not supported by later experience.

The unipolar method is commonly used, the laryngeal electrode being attached to the cathode. The
current varies from 20 to 50 milliamperes, beginning
with the weaker current and gradually increasing as
the patient becomes accustomed to the applictions.

Each treatment should last from one to three
minutes.

The pain is considerable even after thorough cocainization.

CHAPTER XIV.

SURGICAL TREATMENT.—EXTRALARYNGEAL OPERATIONS.

TRACHEOTOMY.

In cases of advanced laryngeal tuberculosis with incipient or no demonstrable pulmonary involvement, tracheotomy is a rational procedure that promises moderately favorable results.

In no case, however, regardless of the conditions, should a tracheal cannula be introduced until all of the less radical methods of treatment have been unavailingly applied.

In four types of the disease the operation may occasionally, though rarely, be indicated.

(1). Advanced laryngeal without pulmonary involvement.

(2). In children so young as to preclude the possibility of successful intralaryngeal treatment.

(3). In cases of extreme and rapidly progressive stenosis.

(4). In certain cases complicated by pregnancy.

Of the curative value of tracheotomy, Moritz Schmidt (*Ueb. Tracheot. b. Kehlkopfschwindsucht D. Med. Woch. Nr.*, 43, 1887) has long been the most ardent advocate, and his views have been endorsed to a certain extent by Chiari, Seifert, Castex, Keimer, Gaudier, Henrici, Beverly Robinson, Finder, Grazzi and others.

Many equally distinguished laryngologists, among whom may be mentioned Hofmann, Lennox Brown, Tietze, Massei, Morrell Mackenzie, B. Fränkel, and Gouguenheim, utterly condemn the procedure.

That the operation exerts a marked, curative effect cannot be questioned in the face of the many reported cases of complete healing and the yet larger number in whom temporary arrest resulted, but the good effects in the majority of instances are more than outweighed by its unfavorable influence upon the pulmonary process.

If the lung condition is perfectly quiescent it may possibly remain so despite the operation, but if there is any activity the wearing of a cannula is almost certain to cause grievous mischief.

It is extremely rare to find advanced laryngeal disease unassociated with active lung lesions, and practically all cases of this so-called "primary" laryngeal phthisis are curable by medicinal or endolaryngeal surgical treatment, so it is a self-evident fact that a question concerning the advisability of tracheotomy almost never arises.

Moritz Schmidt himself made later acknowledgement that the more frequent performance of endolaryngeal operations reduced greatly the number of cases in which he was forced to perform tracheotomy.

The literature shows a large number of reported cures but it will suffice to record one, a typical case, described by Price-Brown (Ann. Otology, Rhinology and Laryngology, June, 1903).

This patient, a man of 30 years, had severe and progressive dyspnea due to enormous infiltration of the epiglottis, completely hiding the arytenoids and vocal cords. One year previous, both his lungs and larynx had shown advanced disease, "considerable deposit in the right apex, extensive consolidation in the left apex, and down the posterior side of the left lung as far as the seventh rib; xxx larynx infiltrated, particularly the left side of the epiglottis. Ulceration along the margin of the left vocal cord, slight abrasion of the left arytenoid and aryepiglottic fold."

At the time of operation his pulmonary condition had greatly improved and expectoration had almost ceased.

In June, seven months after the operation, "the infiltration of the epiglottis has very much diminished; the left side which was so enormously infiltrated has shrunk to less than normal size. There are no visible ulcerations."

Henrici (*Archiv. f. Laryngologie u. Rhinologie*, B. 15, H. 2) reports four successful cases.

Serkowski (Allgem. Med. Chi. Zeitung, Aug., 1878) reported one case alive three years after operation, and Schmidt recorded seven cures.

On the other hand many operators have failed to observe any curative effects whatsoever, for example, Morrell Mackenzie operated twelve cases and in not a single one was there visible improvement in the pathological process.

I have performed the operation five times in all; of these patients two were well after twelve and eighteen months respectively; on died after 11 hours; one succumbed to pulmonary tuberculosis after four months, the larynx having in the meantime showed no recurrence, and one died in seven weeks, the operation having undoubtedly hastened the end.

Of these the first two were cases of moderately advanced laryngeal phthisis with, in both instances, a pulmonary lesion limited to slight consolidation of the right apex, cases that offer a hopeful prognosis from even simple medicinal treatment. The third was a case of sudden abductor paralysis in a young woman with advanced pulmonary and laryngeal tuberculosis. At the time of operation the entire left side was filled with a large pleural effusion.

Both the fourth and fifth cases had moderate and slowly progressive stenosis with fairly widespread pulmonary involvement. In these two cases the pulmonary disease was much aggravated by the operation, and extensive endolaryngeal work would undoubtedly have been the preferable procedure.

The curative effects of tracheotomy depend upon the complete rest given the larynx and upon its protection from irritant dust and pulmonary excretions. Unfavorable results are the rule, however, and are to be credited to some one or more of the following causes:

(1). Aggravation of the lung disease.
(2). Tracheal irritation.
(3). Wound infection.

With a tube in the trachea cough at once becomes weak and ineffectual, the secretions are dammed back in the lungs, fever results, and the entire tuberculous process takes on new activity.

Because of this the performance of tracheotomy must be unqualifiedly condemned except for certain cases in early life, in exceptional pregnancy cases, and in rare instances of acute or rapidly progressive stenosis.

In the so-called primary cases the operation is seldom necessary because other treatment is effective and is attended with little danger, either of local infection or of increased activity in the constitutional malady.

In very young children the difficulty of carrying out effective endolaryngeal treatment makes the operation of tracheotomy a rational and necessary one, even if it be at the risk of increased constitutional disturbance.

Levy (Annals of Otology and Laryngology, Sept., 1906) reports a case of a child tracheotomized by him for laryngeal papillomata. The tube was worn for a considerable period during which the growths were being removed, and the child soon developed and died from tuberculosis. He credited the pulmonary infection to the tracheal opening.

It is certain that the wearing of a cannula irritates the trachea and if its presence favors infection as this case indicates, it would naturally cause increased activity in an already existent lesion.

Tracheotomy even in children should therefore be postponed until the futility of all other treatment has been proven.

In cases of extreme stenosis with rapidly progressive dyspnea an immediate tracheotomy is sometimes required, but early endo-laryngeal surgical management will practically always avert such symptoms and the operation becomes imperative, therefore, only in those cases where treatment has been long neglected.

PREGNANCY.

The mortality in cases of laryngeal tuberculosis complicated by pregnancy is always high no matter what system of treatment is instituted.

Of the seventy-one cases collected by Sokolowski, fifty-six died during or soon after confinement, one was living after eight years and fourteen disappeared.

Of fourteen cases operated by tracheotomy, eleven died, two were lost sight of after discharge and the third was living after eight years.

Three cases were treated by laryngo-fissure; of these two died and one disappeared one month after successful delivery.

Küttner gives the following resumé of 230 pregnant women who had diffuse laryngeal tuberculosis:

"Three survived a natural confinement for one to one and a half years, and thirteen for a longer period, in all, sixteen, or seven or eight per cent.

Among these sixteen women are several in whom the laryngeal affection did not commence until the latter part of the period of gestation. Nearly all surviving subjects belonged to the wealthier classes.

Artifical abortion was induced in twelve cases; in nine with good results, in three without success. Induced premature birth was attempted in seven cases, in one (middle of the seventh month) with, in six without success.

Tracheotomy, or laryngo-fissure respectively, was performed fifteen times. Two of these women survived confinement one to one and one-half years, two still longer, while eleven died soon afterwards. Of these 230 women about 200 died previous to or shortly after confinement, either without professional intervention or notwithstanding it.

Of one hundred and sixteen children concerning whom we have information, seventy-nine or eighty per cent are reported dead; eighteen as living at birth, or in the first two years; nineteen as living a longer time; in all thirty-seven or thirty-two per cent.

In wealthy families the mortality of the children was less than among the poor; likewise do the chances for the child seem better when the mother's life is saved."

Every case of pregnancy complicated by laryngeal tuberculosis should be terminated at the earliest possible moment; if allowed to continue the prognosis is almost hopeless.

If pregnancy is far advanced, however, and the laryngeal infection severe, the induction of abortion will probably hasten the fatal result; in such cases tracheotomy must be at once performed although the hope of a successful issue is slight.

No patient with tuberculosis of the larynx should be allowed to become pregnant but if it does occur the earlier abortion is induced the better the prognosis. If pregnancy is already far advanced when the case comes under observation, tracheotomy is the only recourse.

INTUBATION.

Intubation in laryngeal tuberculosis is wrong in theory and unsuccessful in practice.

Stenosis sufficiently advanced to require radical surgical treatment demands tracheotomy or thyrotomy and not intubation.

The intubation tube acts as an active irritant, causing severe pain, local inflammation, and increase of cough with early expulsion of the tube. Subchordal and chordal lesions alone can be influenced by the tube and disease of these segments rarely leads to serious dyspnea.

The stenosis of tuberculosis is an essentially chronic process (cases of acute tuberculous edema are rare and are responsive to medicinal treatment or to scarification) and tubes of this character can have no permanent influence.

THYROTOMY.

The operation of thyrotomy has not been performed in a sufficient number of cases to definitely establish its true sphere and worth. The results in the comparatively few cases already recorded have not been brilliant, although they have been sufficiently encouraging in a few instances, to warrant the belief that it may be justified in cases of advanced laryngeal with incipient pulmonary disease, provided all other treatment has failed.

A careful review of the literature reveals 43 cases, a considerable proportion of which were operated because of a mistaken or doubtful diagnosis.

Observer	Cases	Deaths	Improvement
Billroth	1	1	..
Dehio	1	1	..
Henning	2	1	1
Schönborn	4	3	2
Hopmann	4	1	3
Küster	2	1	2
Schnitzler	1	..	1
Koch	1	..	1
Grünwald	*2		2
Kijewski	1		1
Baurowicz	1		1
Taptas	1		1
Gerster	1	..	1
Lock	1	..	1
Goris	4	..	4
Bond	†2	..	1
Symonds	‡2		..
Sokolowsky	1		1
Schmiegelow	1		1
Küttner	2		2
Schmidt	2		2
Chavasse	1		1
Gluck	1	..	1
Stein	2	..	2
Lockard	2	1	2
Total	**43**	**9**	**34**

* 1 Unfavorable.   † 1 Unfavorable.   ‡ 2 Unfavorable.

A study of these cases shows that four died soon after operation without laryngeal improvement; five improved locally but died shortly afterwards from the lung disease; four are classed as "unfavorable," and thirty-four improved locally or locally and generally.

Among the improved cases are three that ended fatally but in which the laryngeal symptoms had appreciably lessened.

These statistics are of small value in that the word "improved" means but little, for some temporary betterment is the almost invariable consequence of all treatments, whether surgical or medicinal, in cases where the lung condition is favorable.

The permancy of relief alone offers a standard by which to judge of the comparative effectiveness of the various systems of treatment, and upon this point the records are incomplete.

One of Grünwald's patients showed no signs of recurrence after thirteen months; one of Hopmann's, a preacher, continued to use his voice in public after eleven years; Goris is credited with four cured cases, and Schmidt had one patient still well after six months, and one in whom there was no recurrence at the end of two years.

Otto Stein (Laryngoscope, October, 1904) operated two cases; one showed no signs of return nearly two years after operation, and the other, one year after operation, was cured as to the throat lesion and much improved in general health.

The patient reported by Chavasse lived in comparative comfort for fifteen months.

One of the author's cases, operated in 1901, was living four years later with no subjective symptoms, but the throat had not been examined since a few months after operation. In this case there was widespread laryngeal involvement; great infiltration of both ventricular bands and both arytenoids, with ulceration of the interarytenoid sulcus and the posterior ends of both cords. The pulmonary condition was highly favorable, only slight involvement at the right apex, no temperature and practically no cough or expectoration.

The second case died after five months but the laryngeal lesion had not recurred.

Th. Gluck of Berlin (Annals of Laryngology, Sept., 1904) describes his method of operating and records a case that had no recurrence after seven years. He says:

"In tuberculosis of the larynx and epiglottis, where an extensive surgical operation is required, I pursue the following technique: Total laryngo-fissure, exenteration of the larynx, with excision of diseased cartilage, extirpation of the epiglottis, as a final step, free use of the cautery, then iodoform tamponade of the wound and the insertion of a canula. The patients can swallow after this operation without the slightest difficulty.

After about eight days, a little of the cartilage is resected from the fissure of the thyroid and cricoid cartilages.

Total laryngoplasty, using pedunculated flaps, or, where possible, bridge flaps, and fixing them to the mucous membrane of the pyriform sinus, and to the lateral and posterior aspects of the trachea by means of accurately applied sutures.

One or two sutures also fix the flaps in the depth of the laryngeal cavity. Preferably these flaps are taken from the submental region. If the patient has a beard we must take the flaps form a hairless part of the face. The flaps are also partly secured by iodoform packings. After healing occurs, the patient has an artificial laryngoschism which, however, does not interfere with speech, because the two edges of the thyroid cartilage come together. By these plastic operations one can fill out the whole laryngeal cavity with skin grafts and this skin takes on the character of mucous membrane.

I performed this operation for the first time seven years ago, with excellent results, on a young merchant.

He still remains in perfect health. I had removed one of his testicles for caseous tuberculous orchitis and epididymitis. He suffered from pulmonary tuberculosis, with severe dysphagia and dyspnea.

In this case I may claim with perfect right, that by means of total laryngoplasty, I formed a new larynx for him. The patient does not wear a canula, but breathes through his laryngo-fissure, seems perfectly well, and attends to business.

He speaks in a loud tone of voice, which he can modify, and he can sing the notes of the scale. His cutaneous aditus laryngis is an elliptical slit, about twice the size of a split pea; and thanks to the fact that the expired air causes the free edges of this slit to vibrate, he can speak excellently well and loud. Had the slit been too wide he would at most have been able to whisper. In other words we here have a case of laryngeal tuberculosis, treated as a local tuberculosis, and as a result, permanent healing was secured."

The patient operated by Taptas was much improved in general health, and showed no signs of local recurrence, two and one-half months after operation.

Other so-called cures are recorded but the data is insufficient for conclusive deductions.

Goris, in a compilation of 14 cases, records nine deaths within six months of operation, four complete cures, and one death where the larynx was cured, but the patient died after two years from pulmonary tuberculosis.

Thus while the statistics show a fair number of enduring cures, the fact must not be overlooked that the type of disease for which the operation is peculiarly qualified is one that will respond equally well, and usually much better, to simple medicinal, or at most, to radical endolaryngeal surgical treatment.

Thyrotomy is absolutely contraindicated in cases of advanced pulmonary disease and in those with active lesions no matter how circumscribed. It may, perhaps, be occasionally justifiable in cases of slight pulmonary involvement associated with far advanced laryngeal disease, but only in case the laryngeal condition has been steadily progressive despite radical endo-laryngeal surgical treatment.

Such cases are exceedingly rare.

Thyrotomy, like tracheotomy, usually stimulates the pulmonary process into renewed activity, hence extreme care in the selection of cases for operation is essential.

As a pure palliative procedure the operation is unwarranted, for more certain relief is afforded by other and less dangerous methods.

LARYNGECTOMY.

All observers agree that total excision of the larynx for tuberculosis is never permissible.

If one had to deal simply with an advanced, primary infection the question would be entirely different, but probably without exception the laryngitis is secondary to foci in other organs, usually of the lungs, and complete eradication of the disease in therefore impossible.

The operation has been performed a number of times, (Gussenbauer, Kocher, and Lloyd) and generally because of having mistaken the tuberculous for a carcinomatous growth.

The mortality from laryngectomy, whatever the nature of the disease, is exceedingly high, and it is especially so in tuberculosis where the general condition is usually poor.

Increased activity in the lungs is an invariable sequel, and the unfortunate patients' condition, already deplorable, is greatly aggravated.

In certain rare cases of thyroid perichondritis a partial removal may be necessary but complete excision is to be unqualifiedly condemned.

CHAPTER XV.

THE NOSE.

The entrance of tubercle bacilli into the mucous membrane of the nose may be followed by the development of one of two groups of phenomena, the tuberculous or the lupoid.

Clinically the two processes are usually distinct but their practical identity must nevertheless be admitted: they develop from the same bacillus, their symptomatology differs but little and that largely in virulence or intensity, and their histologic structure shows variations in grade of development only, not in type.

Independent only in name and certain minor symptomatic and unknown etiologic considerations, a comprehensive discussion of either disease, without embracing the other to a certain extent, is impracticable.

Because of this dual nature the literature is both voluminous and to a certain extent misleading, many observers having maintained the absolute identity of the two processes, while others persisted in classifying them as distinct pathologic entities.

Even in many modern case reports it is impossible to determine definitely which of the two conditions actually existed.

HISTORICAL SURVEY.

Lupus of the external nose was described as early as the year 1798 (Willan, Cutaneous Diseases), but its occurrence upon the intra-nasal mucosa was not recorded until fifty years later, when Cazenave ((a). *Abégé;* (b). *Mém. s. l. Coryza Chron.*, 1847-1848) gave the following description:

"Frequently this form of lupus begins upon the nasal mucous membrane, and in this locality extends with unusual rapidity, sometimes until the entire septum is destroyed before ulceration begins upon the skin surface. On the other hand it may bore through the floor of the nose, extend forward upon the palate, and form deep grooves in the gums."

The first authentic observation of a true tuberculous lesion of the nose—a septal ulcer—appears to have been made by Willigk, in 1856 (*Prag. Vierteljahrsschr. f. prakt. Heilk*, 13 *Jahrgang*), the result of 476 autopsies upon tuberculous cadavers.

From this time a full score of years elapsed before record was made of the first definite case of tuberculosis, apart from lupus, seen in the living body.

The virtual identity of the two diseases had, however, already been suspected, for in 1874 Friedländer (*Untersuchungen ueber Lupus,* Virchow's Arch., Bd. 60) maintained that they were identical processes, on the ground of like histologic structure.

The later discovery of the tubercle bacillus, its demonstration in lupoïd as well as in tuberculous tissue, and the results of inoculation tests definitely confirmed Friedländer's suppositions.

In 1877 Laveran (*Un méd. Nr.*, 35-63) described two cases of septal ulceration in patients with pulmonary and laryngeal tuberculosis, and microscopic examination showed tubercles and giant cells in both instances.

In the following year Riedel (*Deutsche Zeitschr. f. Chir., Bd.* 10) reported two additional nasal cases, both of which were apparently primary.

An entirely new type of lesion was described by Thornwaldt in 1880 (*Deutsche Arch. f. Klin. Med., Bd.* 77): A man of 26 years, with hereditary taint, had tuberculosis of the lungs, larynx and pharynx, and the left nostril contained a small tuberculus tumor on the anterior end of the inferior turbinate, and a similar but somewhat smaller growth on the floor of the nose. The posterior end of the septum was ulcerated and the mucous membrane over the cartilaginous portion was studded with granulations similar to those surrounding the tumors.

That neither tuberculosis nor lupus was frequently recognized at this period, however, is witnessed by the writings of Michel, Fränkel, and Mackenzie.

Michel (*Die Krankheiten der Nasenhöhle*, pg. 47, 1876) claimed that he had never seen a case of ulceration of the nose that was not dependent upon syphilis, while both Mackenzie (Diseases of the Nose and Throat) and Heryng (*V. Zeimssen's Handbuch, Bd.* 5, H. I.) asserted that they had never seen a single case of nasal tuberculosis.

Additional cases by Tornwaldt (*Deutsche Zeitschr. f. Klin. Med., Nr.* 27, 1880); Weichselbaum (*Allg. Wien. Med. Ztg. Nr.* 27-28, 1881); Milliard (*Soc. Méd. des Hôp.*, 1881) and Riehl (*Wien med. Woch. Nr.* 44, 1881) were soon reported, but no case departing from the already described types was recorded until Demme (*Z. diagnost. Bedeut. d. Tuberkelbacillen f. d. Kindesalter, Berlin. Klin. Wochenschrift, Nr.* 15, 1883), in a description of two patients, drew attention to the occasional coincidence of tuberculosis and ozena.

One of these cases, a child of twelve months, had "ozena scrofulosa," and later developed and died from pulmonary tuberculosis.

The other, a baby of eight months, developed ozena two months after its adoption into a family the father of which had pulmonary tuberculosis. The septum showed a small ulcer surrounded by minute grayish yellow nodules. Death was due to meningitis tuberculosa and autopsy proved all the other organs to be free from the disease. Bacilli and giant cells were found in the nasal mucosa.

Before this communication, Volkmann (*Tuberculose Erkrankungen der dem Chirurgen zugänglich in Schleimhäute, Beiblatt. z. Centralbl. f. Chirurgie, Nr.* 24, and *Centralb. für Chirurgie, Nr.* 3, 1882) had advanced the theory of a tuberculous ozena dependent upon true tuberculous ulceration of the nose, and maintained that it was absolutely distinct from the much more frequent "Rhinitis scrofulosa" which depended upon simple catarrhal inflammation.

The fact that tuberculous fibromata are a frequent form of intra-nasal tuberculosis was brought forward by König in 1885, and his observations have been amply supported by subsequent statistics.

So many cases were now recorded in quick succession that by 1887 Cartaz (*D. l. Tuberculose nas.* France

Medicale) was able to collect eighteen cases in addition to one of his own.

He classified nasal tuberculosis under two heads: tumor-like growths generally primary, and ulcers, dependent usually upon preceding disease elsewhere. The two varieties may coexist.

Two years later, Hajek (*D. Tuberculose d. Nasenschleimhaut*, 1889) brought forward twenty-seven cases and added thereto three of his own, and in the following year Plicque found forty published cases.

The latter author divided the tuberculous lesions into three groups: granulations, ulcerations and tumors.

Heryng (*Tuberculose d. Nasenschleimhaut*, 1892) assembled ninety cases, and in 1895 Störk (*Die Erkankungen der Nase, Nothnagel's Spec. Path. u. Therapy*, Bd. 13, I Theil) added twenty new patients.

It can avail little to record all subsequent cases and while the number increases more rapidly as we become more diligent in studying all tuberculous patients, nasal tuberculosis can never be considered as other than the rarest form of infection in the respiratory tract.

Up to this time no reference is found bearing upon tuberculous involvements of the accessory sinuses, but in 1889, Demme (27 *Bericht des Jennerschen Kinderhospitals, Bern.*) reported an interesting case of maxillary sinus disease. In this case a nurse, who had a chronic dental fistula with purulent discharge and septal lupus, was responsible for the development of fatal primary intestinal tuberculosis in four children, all of whom had non-tuberculous parents, through her practice of tasting all food before administering it to her charges.

Curettement and irrigations caused eventual healing.

In the following decade a number of additional cases were placed upon record by Rethi (*Wiener Med. Presse*, May 7, 1893); (*Ibid*, No. 51, 1899); Maydl (*Weiner klin. Wochenschrift*, No. 51, 1899); Killian (*Münchener Med. Wochenschrift*, No. 4, 5, 6, 1892); Zander (*Empyema Antri Highmori Dissertatio*, Halle, 1894); Newmayer (*Arch. f. Laryngologie*, II, 1895); Keckwick (*British Journal of Dental Science*, May 13, 1895); Dmochowski (*Arch. f. laryngologie*, III, 1895); Grünwald (*Die Lehre von dem Naseneiterungen*, München, 1896); E. Fränkel (*Virchow's Archiv*. Vol. 143, 1896) and Gaudier (*Rev. Hebd. de Laryngol*. No. 44, 1897).

The cases of Gaudier and Keckwick were apparently of a primary nature.

Involvements of the frontal sinus were recorded by four observers only: Vohsen (*Verhandlungen des X Internationalen Medizinischen Congresses*, Berlin, 1890, Vol. IV, Part 12); Franks and Kunze (*New York Medical Record*, Nov. 3, 1894); Schenke (*Dissertatio*, Jena, 1898) and Panse (*Arch. f. Laryngologie*, XI, 1901).

The case described by Panse, in addition to the frontal and maxillary disease, had extensive involvement of the ethmoid and sphenoid cells.

Hahn (*Ueb. Tuberculose d. Nasenschleimhaut*, D. Med. Wochenschrift, Nr. 23, 1890) in accordance with the majority of clinicians, believed that the form of nasal lesion depended upon the type of infection, i. e., that the tumor represented a primary infection and that the ulcer was invariably secondary.

In the same year Olympitis grouped nasal tuberculosis according to the following types:

1. *Forme aigue.*
2. *Forme chronique.*

1. F. chr. primitive:
   (a) *variété polypoide.*
   (b) *variété infiltrée.*
   (c) *ozène tuberculeux.*
   (d) *abscès tuberculeux.*
   sous-muqueux.

2. *F. chr. secondaire:*
   (a) *forme ulcéreuse.*
   (b) *forme caséeuse.*

The **acute miliary, the ulcerous, and** the caseous varieties **represent secondary, the remaining** types, primary infections.

To this classification Gerber (Heymann's *Handbuch der Laryngologie, 3 Band,* 10 *Lieferung, Seite,* 915) made objection on the ground that only one case of acute nasal infection is recorded; that the existence of an "ozena tuberculosa" is not indisputably proven, and because the types classed as "*abscès tuberculeux*" and "*forme caséeuse*" are founded upon single observations in each case and, moreover, that they are not distinct forms but merely subdivisions of clearly defined types. He substituted the following classification:

1. The tuberculous ulcer.
2. The tuberculous tumor.
3. The diffuse infiltrate. } Lupus.
4. The granulating type. }

Since the two conditions are practically identical, Massei (*Revue hebdomadaire de Laryngologie,* March 11, 1905) proposed that the name lupus be entirely done away with and that all the conditions coming under the two heads be known as tuberculosis.

The last word upon this subject of differentiation, in which a position diametrically opposed to Massei's was taken, is quoted from the article by Henri Caboche which appeared in the Annales des Maladies de l'Orville of October, 1907.

He says: "We see then, to sum up, that there exist only two varieties of nasal tuberculosis: Miliary tuberculosis with frank and unequivocal characteristics, and lupus which comprises: tubercular tumors and the majority of tubercular vegetations."

"The facts seem to me clearly demonstrated: Under the names of tuberculous tumor, vegetating tuberculosis and lupus, writers have described a sole and single thing. This identical thing should be called lupus, for it is characterized objectively and functionally by the same symptoms which, as I have shown already, characterize pituitary manifestations of those having skin lupus."

ETIOLOGY.

In view of the ubiquity of the tubercle bacillus, considerable numbers must occasionally be drawn into the nasal cavities of nearly all healthy individuals, and still more must this be the case with consumptives.

Under normal conditions but few pass into the nasopharynx and from there into the deeper parts of the respiratory tract, for the nose so perfectly performs its function as a filter that only an exceedingly small proportion of the air-contained micro-organisms, no matter what their character may be, penetrate beyond the introitus, and owing to some peculiar property of the nasal cavities and secretions, these rarely exert any baneful effects.

That the mucus of a considerable percentage of healthy individuals contains bacilli has been shown by numerous investigators:

Strauss examined the nasal secretions of 29 persons employed in rooms inhabited by consumptives, and found virulent tubercle bacilli in nine.

Jones (Medical Record, Aug. 25, 1900) injected guinea pigs with mucus from the nostrils of average healthy persons not associated with consumptives, and had positive results in 10.3 per cent of the cases.

Single bacilli must frequently be deposited upon the anterior part of the cartilaginous septum, the point where the inspired air first impinges, and particularly must this be the case in consumptives where, in addition to the ordinary route of inhalation, they may be introduced by infected handkerchiefs and fingers.

Despite the frequent deposit of bacilli at this point, however, and their proven ability to penetrate gland ducts and intact mucous membranes, infection is much rarer than in any other portion of the respiratory tract. The total number of cases recorded does not greatly exceed 150.

In 1901 Knight was able to find but 108 reported cases.

The relative proportion of nasal to pulmonary and laryngeal cases is shown in the following table:

Author	Cases		Nasal Tuberculosis
Weichselbaum	146	consumptive cadavers	2
Willigk	476	consumptive cadavers	1
E. Fränkel	50	consumptive cadavers	0
Schmalfuss	1287	consumptives	0
Henry Phipps Institute	389	consumptives*	0
Steward	2777	nose and throat cases	3
Gerber	1052	nose and throat cases	10
Schäffer	450	nasal tumors	8
Delavan	114	local tuberculosis	5
Lockard	904	local tuberculosis	9
	7645		38

*158 Laryngeal Cases.

Thus, 3366 consumptives (672 cadavers) showed only 17 cases of nasal tuberculosis, and among 4279 nose and throat cases there were but 21 with tuberculosis of the nose.

Of the accessory sinuses, in so far as reliable statistics are available, the maxillary has been tuberculous some twenty-two times, the frontal cells in four cases, and the ethmoidal and sphenoidal combined in two cases.

While it cannot be denied that this form of infection is extremely rare, it is probably much less infrequent than these statistics indicate.

The lesion may easily be overlooked because of its sluggish course and the greater importance of other symptoms, or it may be mistaken for simpler conditions because of its obscure symptomatology and history, yet despite the many probable omissions, nasal infection cannot be considered as other than the rarest form of respiratory tuberculosis.

The deposit of bacilli has been shown to lessen progressively from the nasal introitus to the lungs, yet the frequency of infection increases in inverse ratio: first the lungs, then the larynx, the pharynx, and finally the nose.

Since infection is rarest at the point naturally most exposed to infection, one must assume for the nasal mucous membrane or its secretions some strong inherent power of defense, for the theory of an absence of predisposition to tuberculosis is untenable in view of the fact that a large number of individuals who successfully resist nasal infection fall prey to pulmonary tuberculosis, and that in some of these patients nasal infection occurs later on.

What, then, are these means of defense?

First in importance ranks the peculiar character of the nasal secretion which renders it antagonistic to the life or growth of morbific germs.

Würtz and Lermoyez have shown that even the most resitant of anthrax spores are killed by the nasal mucus within three hours, and E. L. Shurly has proved that this antitoxic property is not peculiar to man but is also present in the mucus of monkeys.

Liaras, and Park and Wright, do not fully accept these views as to the bactericidal power of the mucus but admit that it is an exceedingly poor culture medium.

Experiments made by St. Clair Thompson and Hewlitt prove unmistakably that bacteria cannot thrive within the nostrils. In one group of experiments pure cultures of the Bacillus Prodigiosus were placed upon the anterior part of the septum, and after fifteen minutes there was found to be a considerable diminution in the number of bacteria; after eighty minutes none could be found and at the end of two hours no growth could be obtained in cultures.

In the second series a measured quantity of laboratory air, containing 29 mould spores and nine bacteria, was passed through the nose and measured as it passed through the choanae, and was found to have lost all but two of the mould spores and all of the bacteria.

Piaget claims that the nasal mucus is absolutely fatal to the anthrax bacillus, the diphtheritic bacillus, the colon bacillus and some forms of the streptococcus and staphylococcus.

The second barrier is formed by the extreme sensitiveness and reflex irritability of the nasal mucous membrane, whereby the inhalation of any irritant provokes almost instantaneous congestion, swelling of the erectile tissues and increased flow of the watery secretions, with probable expulsion of the foreign element. If this proves ineffectual the resultant sneezing and blowing of the nose aid in cleansing the tissues.

The normal flow of the secretions from the roof of the nose downward, and either to the anterior or posterior openings, carries with it nearly all of the extraneous substances, and in this cleansing action the cilia take part.

The bacilli find additional obstacles to premanent lodgement in the constant presence of a film of protective mucus, in the filtering functions of the vibrissae and in the character of the tissues at certain points, i. e., squamous epithelium.

This combination of defensive agencies is generally sufficient to repel any injurious invasion but it may prove unavailing, *first,* when large numbers of bacilli are introduced at one time and *secondly,* when by reason of previous or simultaneous disease, or traumatism, one or more of the barriers are weakened or destroyed.

Demonstrating the effect produced by the simultaneous introduction of a large number of bacilli, the following experiments may be cited:

De Bono and Frisco (*Annali d' Igiene Sper.*, 1901-03) produced tuberculosis in guinea pigs by inoculation with the aqueous humor of the eyes of rabbits, aspirated one hour after pure cultures of tubercle bacilli were brought into contact with the nasal mucous membranes.

Renshaw (Journal of Pathology, 1901), by applying bacilli to the uninjured nasal mucosa, produced tuberculosis of the lymphatic glands in seven of eight cases.

Cornet obtained similar results, introducing the bacilli upon a pigeon feather in order to avoid traumatism.

While, in rare instances, the bacilli may penetrate an intact epithelial surface, some previous disease or traumatism is usually essential. Perhaps the most frequent contributory factor is the condition known as Xanthosis. The inspiratory air current first strikes the cartilaginous septum and there deposits a considerable part of its contained dust and micro-organisms. The irritation from, and the separation of, this dust scab produce erosions, with hemorrhage and degeneration. In many cases the traumatism results from forcible blowing or picking of the nose and these habits are therefore especially reprehensible in consumptives. It is upon this spot that nasal tuberculosis usually originates.

Both the ulcer and tumor occur most frequently within this damaged area; in Steward's collection of 100 cases the septum was attacked in 89 per cent, and was the sole nasal localization in 70 per cent.

The traumatism may result in subsequent inhalation infection or what is more probable, simultaneous infection by means of bacilli already present in the nose or deposited soon afterward by infected finger-nails and handkerchiefs. Schmitthuisen (Journal of Laryngology, Pg. 397, 1900) and Kiar (*Rev. de Laryngol.*, Pg. 263, 1901) have recorded cases which seem to have been produced in this way, and Schech (*Krankheiten der Mundhöhle, Pg.* 316-317, 1896) describes the case of a woman who acquired nasal tuberculosis by using the unwashed handkerchief of her tuberculous husband.

It is a common practise to ascribe to catarrh a prominent place in etiology because of the resultant abrasions and lessened vitality of the mucosa. It has been conclusively demonstrated, however, that catarrhal inflammations markedly reduce the absorptive properties of the tissues and this factor, in connection with the diminished caliber of the nasal cavities and the greatly increased flow of mucus, may fully counteract the effect of the surface erosions.

Hahn has recorded a case of tuberculous tumor in a patient who had a long standing eczema of the upper lip and nose.

Primary and Secondary Infection:—Tuberculosis of the nose may be either primary or secondary, the latter representing the more frequent form of the disease. This is what would naturally be expected from a study of the predisposing causes.

Aside from the not infrequent conveyance of infection through the lymph channels and blood current, the careless consumptive is constantly exposed to the danger of auto-infection by unclean fingers, linen, spray tubes, &c.

Suppressed coughing or violent attacks of retching and vomiting may likewise carry virulent colonies of bacilli into the nasal cavities, and their susceptibility to large numbers of bacilli simultaneously introduced has already been shown.

The introduction of bacilli into the nose by incompletely expectorated sputum was claimed by Kossel to be responsible for the numerous tubercle bacilli found in the nasal mucus of a young girl dead of pulmonary and cerebral tuberculosis. The nasal mucous membranes were found at autopsy to be entirely normal.

In consumptives we also find an occasional transference of the disease from neighboring structures to the nose. Newmayer (*Arch. f. Laryng., Bd.* II, 2 *Heft,* 5260, 1894) records a case in which the nasal lesion could be traced back through the maxillary sinus to a buccal tuberculosis, consequent upon the extraction of a tooth. A similar case is recorded by Rethi (*Wien. Med. Pr.* 19, 1893).

Infection may also occur through palatal perforations (pg. 357).

The comparative frequency of primary and secondary cases depends upon the interpretation of the terms "primary" and "secondary."

If by primary disease is understood all cases in which at the time the nasal lesion becomes manifest no other focus is clinically demonstrable, the disproportion between the two types is not great, but as is the case with the larynx, the primary nature of a lesion cannot be definitely proven except upon the cadaver.

Apparently sound individuals may conceal latent foci that under the influence of trauma will give rise to disseminated infections, that may to all appearances be primary localizations.

The apparently primary lesion, however, is not uncommon. Herzog (Amer. Journal of Med. Sc., Dec., 1893) assembled twenty primary cases to sixty of a secondary nature, and in 1890 Olympitis (*Tubercul. d. l. muqueuse. nas. Thèse*, Paris) found nineteen cases of primary and four of possibly primary origin in a total of thirty-nine cases.

Beermann (*Ueb. prim. Tuberc. d. Nasenschleimh. Diss., Würzburg*, 1890), of twenty-nine cases collected by him, considered ten as probably primary.

Sixteen of twenty-one cases reported by Chiari were primary, and in Steward's collection of one hundred cases, fifty-eight appeared to be primary.

On the other hand, Gonguenheim and Glover (*Atlas de Laryngologie et de Rhinologie*) consider the greater number to be secondary.

Of eight cases of tuberculous nasal tumors seen by Schäffer, none had other demonstrable signs of the disease. Chiari (*Ueb. Tuberculome d. Nasenschleimhaut, Arch. f. Laryngologie*, 1893, *Bd.* I, *Heft*, II, *S*, 121) assembled a total of twenty-one cases of which the following classifications was made:

CASES 22.

Pulmonary Tuberculosis .... 5 cases.
Scrofulous or hereditary taint................ 7 cases.
No demonstrable pulmonary disease..........13 cases.
Evident infection from without.............. 6 cases.
Bacilli found in ....11 cases.
Histologic diagnosis in..................... 6 cases.
Clinical diagnosis only .... 4 cases.

In twenty-two cases of maxillary sinus tuberculosis,
three (Gaudier, Coakley, Keckwick) were without other
evidences of the disease.

We are yet in the dark regarding the *modus operandi*
by which lupus results in one individual and tuberculosis in another.

Lupus, in contradistinction to tuberculosis, is always
a local disease, the result of direct infection of an
abraded skin or mucous membrane and in a large majority of the cases seems to be dependent upon the existence of a strongly marked tuberculous diathesis.

According to Moure it often follows a strumous
pseudo-atrophic coryza.

Sachse (*Beitrag. zur Statistick des Lupus, Viertel-
jahrisch.. f. Derm. u. Syph., Bd.* 13, *S.* 241) found definite signs of tuberculosis or hereditary tendency in
55.89 per cent of all cases; Demme in 37.2 per cent and
Bloch in 25.5 per cent.

Bender (*Ueber die Beziehungen des Lupus vulg. zur
Tuberculose, Berl. Klin. Woch., Nr.* 23-24, 1886), in
159 lupoid patients, found definite signs of tuberculosis
in 109, while Raudnitz found only ten per cent with
hereditary taint.

Bloch claims that three-fourths of all lupoid patients
show other signs of tuberculosis, and he saw eight of
nine such individuals die of pulmonary tuberculosis.

Sachse saw a similar result in six or seven patients.

From a study of a large series of cases Caboche arrives at the following conclusions: "In a certain number of cases the lupus patient does not get well and dies of pulmonary tuberculosis. I have seen this eventuality once. Thus, while the patient with pulmonary tuberculosis never, so to speak, becomes lupic, the reverse is far from rare. (Lenglet)."

Primary lupus of the mucous membranes is comparatively frequent, although it is usually secondary to lupus of the skin.

CASES OF LUPUS.

Observer	Primary in Nasal Mucosa
Caboche	22
Raudnitz	4
Pontoppidan	100
Cozzolino	5
Bloch	10
Bender	75
Mummenhoff	37
Total	253

Many of the more recent observers (Escat, Bresgen, Chiari, Audry, Sticker, Caboche) believe that the majority of cases of facial lupus are secondary to lesions of the mucosa, unobserved because of their sluggish, symptomless course, and transmitted through the lymphatic system.

SEX AND AGE.

Nasal lupus occurs most frequently in women.

Observer	Men	Women
Raudnitz	37.7 %	62.7 %
Pontoppidan	34.0 %	66.0 %
Bloch	31.9 %	68.1 %
	34.4 %	65.6 %

In twenty personal cases of Caboche, eighteen were women and two men.

The relationship is practically the same as in nasal tuberculosis.

Steward in 100 cases found..........41%   59%
Störk in 20 cases found.............20% ,   80%

A comparative study shows:

Lupus 34.4%   65.6%
Tuberculosis 30.5%   69.2%

The age incidence in nasal and laryngeal tuberculosis varies but little.

OZENA AND TUBERCULOSIS.

While not strictly related to the question of the etiology of nasal tuberculosis, the relationship of nasal atrophy to pulmonary tuberculosis is of sufficient importance to merit brief comment.

Demme (*Z. diagnost. Bedeut. d. Tuberkelbacillen f. d. Kindersalter, Ber. Klin. Woch., Nr.* 15, 1883) first drew attention to this relationship by his report of a case of a twelve months old baby that suffered from "ozaena scrofulosa," which later developed and died from pulmonary tuberculosis. Since this report the relationship has been frequently observed and commented upon.

Freudenthal, in an examination of 340 patients of the Bedford Sanatorium for Consumptives (N. Y. Med. Journ., Dec. 19, 1903), found that 115 had a dry condition of the nose or a genuine atrophic condition, and reached the conclusion that, "the dry atrophic condition of the nose and throat produced by our unhygienic system of heating is one important factor in laying the foundation for tuberculosis."

Clark found some evidence of a nasal atrophy in 73 of 170 phthisical patients, and J. K. Hamilton, in 170 cases of ozena, found six with phthisis. A. Alexander (*Arch. f. Laryngologie, B.* 14, *H.* 2) found 31 cases of atrophy in 200 consumptives and 22 cases of tuberculosis in 50 ozena patients. Of the remaining 28 ozena cases, four had other diseases of the lungs and seven were classed as "suspicious."

In 22 autopsies upon ozena patients, phthisis was demonstrated in 15.

Three hundred and eighty-nine consumptives of the Henry Phipps Institute (Second Annual Report) showed six with nasal atrophy.

C. H. Theisen (*Laryngoscope*, Oct., 1904) reported 40 personal cases of ozena; of these 14 had well marked pulmonary tuberculosis.

Liaras (*Thèse de Bordeaux*, 1899) found but two cases of tuberculosis in 52 of ozenatous rhinitis.

The author, in 275 consumptives, met with 49 cases of nasal atrophy.

A summary of these reports shows:

```
1304 Consumptives  ........274 cases of atrophy..........20.25%
 312 Ozena cases.......... 44 consumptives ..............14.1%
```

These statistics make the conclusion irresistible that ozena predisposes to tuberculosis, although the fact must not be lost sight of that in some of these cases the converse may obtain, i. e., the malnutrition antedating the development of tuberculosis or following its advent, may provoke the intra-nasal degeneration.

It has been shown that the nasal mucous membrane and its mucus have certain properties that render the nose unfavorable to the lodgment and development of morbific germs, and it is evident that these barriers are absolutely destroyed by ozena. As Alexander says: "The nose, or the filter which should protect the body from the bad results of the invasion of micro-organisms, itself becomes a permanent source of infection."

Whether or not there is a form of nasal tuberculosis worthy of the designation ozenous is disputed but a careful examination of the so-called confirmatory cases, together with certain theoretical considerations, would tend to the belief that in these patients there has been merely an accidental association of the two conditions, rather than that the ozena depended upon the presence of the tubercle bacilli.

In the few authentic cases recorded in which ozena accompanied tuberculous lesions, the latter were invariably in the form of numerous minute ulcers and since it is a well substantiated fact that ulcerations never occur in true atrophic rhinitis, the belief is warranted that in these patients the tuberculosis was grafted upon tissues already affected by true ozena.

If the bacilli were capable of provoking ozena, is it not surprising, in view of the large number of carefully observed cases of nasal tuberculosis, that not more than three cases have been observed in which this symptom was present?

It has been shown that over 20 per cent of all consumptives, studied with a view of determining the relationship between atrophy and pulmonary tuberculosis, have shown such a condition of the nasal mucosa, hence we have all the conditions most favorable for

PLATE XVII.

FIG. 65. Incipient tuberculosis of the nose, involving the anterior end of the inferior turbinate, the quadrangular cartilage and floor.

FIG. 66. Tuberculous infiltration and ulceration of the posterior portion of the septum and of the pharyngeal tonsil.

PLATE XVII.

FIG. 65. Incipient tuberculosis of the nose.

FIG. 66. Tuberculosis of the posterior septum and the pharyngeal tonsil.

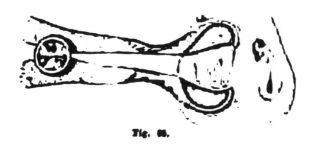

Fig. 65.

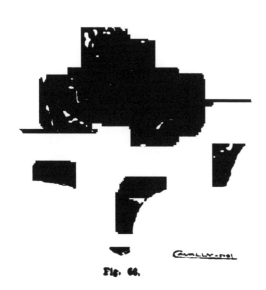

Fig. 66.

PLATE XVII.

infection by both the micro-organisms of ozena and the bacillus of tuberculosis.

SYMPTOMATOLOGY.

Tuberculosis of the nose usually becomes manifest either as a tumor or an ulcer but in very rare instances it may be seen in the stage of circumscribed or diffuse infiltration.

The diffuse infiltrate, however, can scarcely be looked most frequent manifestation of lupus and is generally upon as a typical lesion, because in the nose it is the indicative of a lupoid rather than of a true tuberculous infection. The same may be said of the granuloma.

The ulcer is invariably found in individuals already suffering from other and well-advanced tuberculous processes, usually of the lungs, or lungs and larynx, but the tumor is not infrequently the first and only recognizable focus.

The tumor occurs less frequently than the ulcer although the disparity is not great: the former was met 42 times and the latter 48 times in a total of 90 cases. Of 20 cases seen by Störck, 6 were tumors and 14 ulcers.

As has already been shown, however, both conditions are extremely rare, but 14 cases having been seen in 2694 consumptives, while examination of 672 tuberculous cadavers revealed but three tuberculous lesions of the nose.

Systematic examination of every consumptive would without doubt materially increase the percentage of cases (one case in every one hundred of laryngeal tuberculosis was seen by the author) for in but few patients are the evoked symptoms sufficient to occasion comment, especially when the pulmonary and laryngeal foci are far advanced.

The forms designated as nodular, vegetating, and in-filtrative, because they conform to the appearances usually found in association with facial lupus, are frequently classed as lupic rather than as tuberculous, but as the various types frequently coexist and are to all intents identical processes, they will be so considered and grouped under the common name of tuberculosis. No attempt at strict differentiation will be made, for it can lead only to confusion except in the question of prognosis, where the lesions of a definite lupic character certainly offer a more hopeful prospect than those which conform to the appearances of tuberculosis seen elsewhere.

THE TUMOR.

The tumor, like the ulcer and the infiltrate, attacks by preference the quadrangular cartilage but in rare instances may be primarily situated upon one of the turbinal bodies or the floor of the nose.

When the middle turbinate is involved the case is exceptional, and the inferior body is the primary site in not more than one case in four or five. Invasion of the nasal floor almost never occurs except through extension from the septum or the turbinals and either of these parts may be involved by the process spreading across the floor from one side to the opposite one.

Mercier (*Revue hebdomadaire de Laryngologie*, June 14, 1902) observed a case of tuberculoma in which the posterior end of the septum was alone involved.

When extensive distribution has once occurred, the point of origin can rarely be determined.

The tumor, like its laryngeal prototype, may be single, as is usually the case, or there may be two or more. Many cases classified as tumors have probably not been such at all if the term be understood to designate only those growths that are not preceded by ulceration.

Particularly is this the case with multiple growths, unless they are sharply defined and separated by areas of normal tissue, for the majority of these tumors are merely masses of exuberant granulations springing from and completely hiding underlying ulcers.

The true tuberculoma varies in size from a pea to a small, chicken's egg, and while it is generaly a solid growth it may be composed of a number of firmly united nodules of small size. The mass is round or irregular in form and usually sessile, although not infrequently pedunculated.

The latter type, when covered by a smooth mucosa, grayish or grayish-red in color, bears some resemblance to a fibroma. The color may vary from this transparent gray to a purplish red and the mucous membrane, instead of being smooth and glistening, may be granular or even warty. The surface is sometimes traversed by prominent blood-vessels.

The growth is generally insensitive and bleeds freely on gentle manipulation.

Free bleeding occurs nearly always with tumors that are soft and friable, although a case is recorded by Hahn in which easily provoked hemorrhages occurred from a growth that was of an unusually firm consistency.

The tuberculoma is generally unilateral in the beginning but as time passes, if it be located upon the septum, the dividing wall gives way and a homogeneous mass protrudes into both nostrils. Although in cases of long standing there is practically always ulceration within or about the base of the tumor, involving, perhaps, the entire cartilaginous septum in the destructive process, the surface may and generally does main-in its integrity for a long time.

en ulceration does begin upon the surface the growth melts away with great rapidity and the for the time being, may be entirely occluded by tuberant granulations. These in turn succumb to ru   i process and soon all evidences of the ation may have vanished, leaving no visible signs aside fom the great, and more or less distinctive, septal destruction.

Miliary tubercles are often seen about the circumference and they occasionally dot the entire surface of the growth.

Instead of one primary growth there are sometimes two or more small tumors, occupying different parts of the cartilaginous septum, and each may lead to a distinct perforation.

The subjective symptoms are slight and frequently masked by those consequent upon the pulmonary or laryngeal lesions. In the beginning there is nothing more than partial nasal obstruction which remains unaccompanied by other symptoms until some superficial ulceration occurs, when the nasal secretions become purulent and somewhat foul. In such cases bleeding occurs at intervals and there is considerable scab formation.

Alterations in the shape of the exterior nose have not been observed except in rare cases. Schäffer reports one in which there was a warty thickening of the entire organ.

Both the tumor and the ulcer may, exceptionally, produce a palatal perforation or extensive necrosis of the nasal bones, with a sinking-in of the bridge, the so-called "saddle nose."

The majority of these cases of so-called tuberculous tumors, 44 in all, are classed by Caboche as lupus, on the ground that they occurred in patients free of pulmonary disease and on section usually failed to reveal bacilli. He considers 29 of these growths to be purely lupic.

THE ULCER.

Although the appearance of an ulcer is nearly always preceded by a stage of infiltration, variably long, this antecedent condition is almost never seen because of the few subjective symptoms evoked.

Many authors speak of a "primary" ulcer. Thus Gerber (*Handbuch der Laryngologie und Rhinologie*, 1899, page 916) says:

"The tuberculous nasal ulcer is very rare. I have seen it several times in consumptives. Frequently enough, however, there is ulceration of the infiltrations and granulations."

Although the occurrence of ulceration without preceding infiltration has been repeatedly affirmed, I believe that there can be no question that every tuberculous ulcer occurs upon an infiltrated tissue. We may here, as in the larynx, have a bacillary infection of a simple ulcer but the so-called true ulcer results from caseation of submucous tubercles.

Owing to the rapid destruction when necrosis has nce begun, it is unusual to find evidences of preceding infiltration but this has occasionally been observed.

The early infiltrate may be covered by a smooth, or what is far more frequent, a nodular mucosa; the latter may be of a simple granular character or so infiltrated by la t tubercles as to be distinctly warty.

The sw   hard an fairly resistant, and as
re is li   t ᵉ·t   ation the color does
art fᵢ ·d   ·mal: it is usually a pale red.
ȷ ᵇ n   rormation the tissue becomes
                    (] ate XVII, Fig. 65.)
                    preferred point of attack,
the turbinals are occasionally primarily involved. The septal swelling may be circumscribed or so diffuse as to involve the entire cartilaginous portion; in the latter instance ulceration rapidly ensues with multiple perforations and wide destruction.

When the nostril is filled with exuberant granulations the almost typical picture of a large tumor is presented. Schech stands alone in describing the lesions as poor in granulation tissue (*Krankheiten der Mundhöhle*, pg. 317).

The ulcer in its earliest stages is rarely seen owing to its unobtrusive symptoms and their complete masking by those dependent upon more important lesions.

As the anterior part of the quadrangular cartilage is the elective point for the infiltrate and tumor, it is con-

PLATE XVIII.

Fig. 67. Incipient tuberculosis of the inferior turbinate and meatus.

PLATE XVIII.

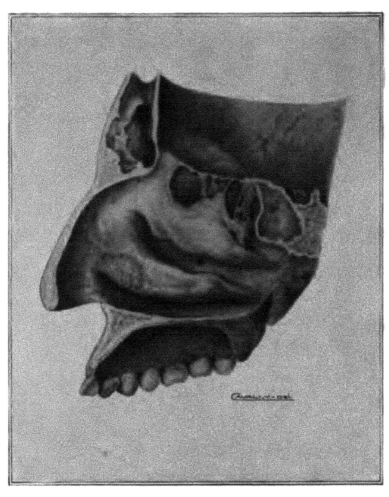

Fig. 67.

sequently the point at which ulceration most often occurs.

The reason for this localization has already been shown to depend upon traumatism and it is at the same point that other traumatic lesions occur, i. e., simple perforating ulcers, occupation necrosis, &c.

From this elective point the process extends across the nasal floor to one or both turbinals, but the transference may occur in the opposite direction from an original focus upon either the inferior or middle turbinal. (Plate XVIII, Fig. 67.)

Pluder (*Zwei Bemerkensw. Fälle v. Tuberculose d. obersten Athmungsw., Arch. f. Laryngologie, Bd., IV, I Heft, S.* 117, 1896) described a case seen by him in which there was widespread ulceration of the posterior edge of the septum and exuberant granulations covering the floor of the nose. In this case the infection occurred through a cleft palate.

Gerber also described a case in which there was wide involvement of and about the choanae. There were numerous miliary tubercles on the vault of the pharynx and the posterior openings were almost obliterated on both sides, on the right by a homogeneous mass, on the left by two distinct tumors. On each side the swelling seemed to spring from the posterior turbinals. The right tube was entirely involved and the left was enormously enlarged and covered with papillomatous excrescences.

Springing from the upper edge of the choana and filling the space between the lateral tumors was a pale teat-like projection of tissue resembling the uvula. The cervical glands were tuberculous and after their ex-

e, surrounded by numerous miliary tu-
small granulations. The surrounding mu-
rane was considerably inflamed. From the
of this ov   middle point,
a narrow, irregular groove extended down the posteri-
or edge of the septum to a point slightly above the lower border. The mucous membrane projected into the
nostrils from each side of the septum and diminished
the normal diameters by about one-half. (Plate XVII,
Fig. 66.) As soon as possible all the diseased tissue was curetted and thoroughly cauter-
ized, and in two months every evidence of the disease had disappeared. He lived for fourteen months
and had no recurrence.

The involvements of the posterior septum and turbinals may originate at these points or extend to them
from contiguous portions of the nose, naso-pharynx
or palate.

The ulcer, when not hidden by granulations, may

have the so-called typical tuberculous characteristics, but on the other hand, owing to frequent bleeding, and irritation and discoloration by the air currents and dust, it may lose these pathognomonic features and be recognized with difficulty.

In the unaltered type we find the same mouse-eaten, irregular edges, uneven base, superficial involvement and grayish or yellowish white discoloration that has been noted in the laryngeal ulcers. Miliary tubercles are occasionally seen in the neighboring tissues and granulations are always present, either projecting from the membranous base or surrounding the ragged edges.

These small projections are generally hidden by a deposit of tenacious muco-pus and come into view only after careful cleansing.

The edges may be considerably undermined and prominent, or even clear cut and infiltrated, and in exceptional cases they merge by gradual transition into an inflamed areola. In some instances the base is perfectly even and appears to be slightly elevated, as though there were a deposit of false membrane. This is due to the breaking down of a tissue already considerably infiltrated.

The ulcers are usually solitary and of variable size and shape—round, oval, serpiginous or irregular.

Two or three separate ulcers occur in some rare cases and a few instances of numerous small ones, dotting the entire septal mucosa, are recorded.

The individual ulcers enlarge through disintegration of surrounding miliary tubercles and the confluence of contiguous spots.

In many cases the initial lesion, whether it be an ulcer, infiltrate or tumor, is entirely hidden by the accompanying granulations, and as already mentioned, these may attain such size and consistency as to closely resemble tuberculomata. As diffuse granulations are almost pathogonomic of lupus, the differential diagnosis, when the nasal lesion is primary, may be exceedingly difficult.

In certain cases, classed usually as lupic, the mucosa is widely studded with small, soft nodules, separated one from the other by irregular grooves and ulcers; in other instances the membrane is extensively thickened with uneven projections and depressions which Caboche describes as follows: "One sees minute hillocks separated by miniature valleys. Each of the hillocks, sometimes rounded like a dome, sometimes terminating in a sharp crest, is made up (the same as the valleys) of an agglomeration of very small nodules the size of a pin head, separated by extremely narrow grooves, giving to the lesion as a whole a muriform aspect which is peculiar to it."

The subjective symptoms are not marked: there is usually slight respiratory obstruction, scab formation and sporadic attacks of bleeding. Pain is not severe and often entirely lacking, and is prominent only when the skin border becomes involved, upon extension of the process to the perichondrium and in cases of acute miliary infection.

Lupus runs a painless course.

Practically all cases advance gradually to perichondritis and chondritis, through direct extension. Primary infection of the bone or cartilage, on the other band, is exceedingly rare. Two such cases have been recorded but in neither was the evidence conclusive.

Perforation of the nasal septum is much more frequent in consumptives than in individuals otherwise normal and while the greater number of these are of simple traumatic origin, a certain proportion depend upon tuberculosis; the edges are not smooth and thin as in the simple variety but enormously thickened, warty and granular. They bleed easily upon manipulation and are generally covered by tenacious scabs of mucus, pus, blood and epithelial cells.

Weichselbaum claims that septal perforations are found twice as often in consumptive as in non-tubeculous cadavers.

According to D. Braden Kyle, septal perforations occur in the proportion of one to every 200 cases of nasal disease, but in the author's series of 904 cases of laryngeal tuberculosis, there were 36 with this condition or one in every 25.

ACCESSORY SINUSES.

As indicated in the Historical review, tuberculosis of the accessory sinuses is a relatively rare condition, the total number of verified cases not exceeding twenty-seven. To this total the maxillary sinus contributed twenty-two; the frontal cells, four; and the ethmoidal and sphenoidal combined, two, one of which is included among the frontal cases as all four sinuses were involved.

Suppurative sinusitis occurs frequently in phthisical patients as is shown by the following table, but there are no figures to indicate how many were tuberculous and how many non-tuberculous.

It is probable that the great majority of these cases did not depend upon the presence of the tubercle bacillus.

Ingersoll and Howard examined a number of cases of chronic suppuration to determine their relationship with tuberculosis but did not find the bacilli in a single instance. In collaboration with Dr. Carmody, the author has examined eight cases of sinusitis occurring in consumptive patients without finding the bacilli in one.

In one post-mortem case, Fränkel found bacilli in a maxillary sinus where tuberculosis had not been diagnosed during life.

From an exhaustive study of twenty published cases of maxillary sinus tuberculosis, Gleitsmann, in an article read before the Twenty-ninth Annual Congress of the American Laryngological Association, drew the following conclusions as to their causation:

"From the histories furnished, we learn, what is to be expected, viz.: that the majority of sinus tuberculosis is due to an extension from a neighboring tuberculous focus. Of the twenty cases of tuberculosis of the maxillary sinus, which I could find, twelve were due to tubercular lesions of the bones of the nose or upper maxilla, whilst in the remaining eight, carious processes of these parts can be excluded. The majority of patients suffered from pulmonary tuberculosis, and a few only had the well-known symptoms of antral empyema without any constitutional disturbances, but at operation tubercle bacilli were found in the discharge evacuated. In eight instances the presence of tubercle bacilli in the antral secretion was verified by microscopical examination.''

In five of these twenty cases the disease reached the sinus by extension from a focus in the alveolar process through a dental fistula.

A case in which the infection travelled in a direction directly opposite to this last described channel was recently seen by the author in consultation with Dr. Carmody.

This patient, a cigar maker, had had pulmonary tuberculosis of several years' duration when the left maxillary sinus became involved. This had been neglected until, after a number of months, pain developed in the incisor with necrosis of the root and loosening of the tooth. The tooth was extracted but shortly afterward a fistula developed and nearly a year elapsed before a cure was effected. The fistula opened above the incisor and extended back of the bicuspid. Tubercle bacilli were not found but the opening in the alveolus was typically tuberculous, as is shown in Fig. 68 and Plate XIX, Fig. 69.

In two of the twenty cases detailed by Gleitsmann infection came from a nasal lupus, in one it occurred through the canine fossa. In all but three of the cases there was pulmonary phthisis.

As a rule it is impossible to demonstrate the presence of tubercle bacilli but this has been done in a small number of instances.

Four cases of frontal sinus tuberculosis have been recorded; in three the frontal was the only cell involved, in one all four sinuses were affected.

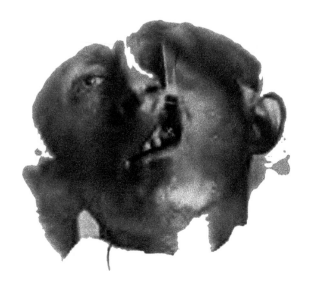

Fig. 68.

These cases were observed by Panse, Franks and Kunze, Vohsen, and Schenke.

Schenke's case, as described by Gleitsmann in the address already referred to, concerned a man 18 years of age who had tuberculosis of the middle ear and cervical glands. "When admitted to the hospital he had a swelling of the frontal region and a fistula of the

PLATE XIX.

Fig. 69.   Perforation of the alveolus due to a tuberculous maxillary empyema.

Fig. 70.   Tuberculous ulceration of the tuberosity.
   (Illustrations used by courtesy of Dr. T. E. Carmody.)

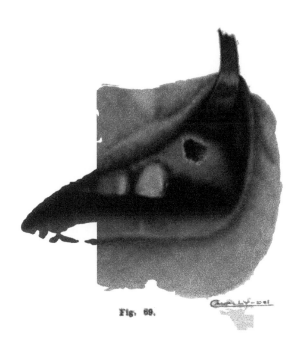

Fig. 69.

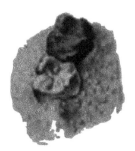

Fig. 70.

PLATE XIX

mastoid process, extending posteriorly towards the cranial basis, and another one leading to the styloid process. A few days after the fistulous ducts had been scraped, the frontal sinus was operated, and tuberculous masses appeared immediately after incision of the skin.

A fistula led to the left sinus, which was thoroughly curetted after complete removal of its anterior wall, and communication with the nose was established. Death took place twelve days after his admission. Postmortem examination showed an abscess of the left mastoid process, extending to the cranial base, and the occipital foramen, into the interior of the cranial cavity, tuberculosis of the frontal sinus, but no perforation into the cranial cavity."

In two of the other cases there was swelling of the frontal region and at operation cheesy masses were found within the sinuses with necrosis of the posterior walls. The third case, Vohsen's, had a fistula leading to carious bone within the sinus.

Two cases of sphenoidal and ethmoidal suppuration of a tuberculous character, in one combined with a like process in the frontal and maxillary sinus, in the other with the maxillary alone, have been observed. The first and more extensive was described by Panse and concerned a young girl of 16 years.

The sphenoidal and frontal sinuses were opened because of a suspicion of involvement of one or the other, on account of a sudden blindness that developed one month after an operation for nasal polypi. Necrotic bone was found in each cell and giant cells were found in the scrapings. Antisyphilitic treatment availed

Fig. 71.

left parietal bone. The optic nerve was destroyed and there was circumscribed meningitis.

The second case was that of a prominent physician who died in Denver in the winter of 1906. He had extensive disease of both lungs and several months before death developed maxillary, sphenoidal and ethmoidal disease on the right side, following a tuberculous infection of the right upper jaw. The corresponding lower jaw rapidly succumbed to the same process after a focus had become established in the region of the first molar. The condition of this alveolus is shown in Fig. 71 and Plate XX, Fig. 72.

The clinical diagnosis and later course of the disease did not permit of any doubt as to the true conditions and the post-mortem gave conclusive evidence as to the cause of the suppuration.

The pathological changes that take place in the sinuses do not vary greatly from those that occur in other structures, hence a separate description is not required.

The prognosis is highly unfavorable; of the cases collected by Gleitsmann three only resulted in temporary cure and nothing is known as to the ultimate outcome. Recurrences are to be anticipated.

Coakley's case was well, both in regard to the local and general condition, one year after the arrest of the maxillary disease; in the author's case the elapsed time is all too short to warrant any definite conclusions.

DIAGNOSIS.

Tuberculosis and syphilis of the nose present striking similarities in their objective appearances and a differential diagnosis, without histologic examination or recourse to the therapeutic test, is often impossible.

In the far advanced lesions we have the fact that tuberculosis usually involves the cartilaginous, and syphilis the bony framework, and that the former, in the majority of cases, is secondary to advanced disease of the lungs and larynx. It must not be forgotten, however, that both diseases may exist in the same individual, that a nasal tuberculosis may occur in one who has syphilis and that syphilis of the nose can occur in one suffering from general tuberculosis.

The formation of large tumors, a common manifestation of tuberculosis, is rare in syphilis.

In the latter disease the subjective symptoms are usually much more severe; there is considerable surrounding inflammation, local and cephalic pain, tenderness on pressure, &c.

The typical variations and classical features of each are detailed on page 132.

In other cases the lupus is accompanied by lacrimation. lymphangitis of the lobule and destruction of the alae.

Between lupus and tuberculosis a strict line cannot be drawn because they are practically identical, depending upon the same cause and differing only in minor clinical characteristics.

Lupus is often associated with lupus of the skin or with a vestibular eczema, and then offers no difficulties in diagnosis.

When primary within the nasal cavities, however, the differentiation may be exceedingly difficult; in general the tuberculous nodules are more sensitive although some cases of tuberculosis are unattended by pain or tenderness. The most significant feature of the tuberculous lesions is the absence of any tendency toward spontaneous arrest. In lupus we find nodules, ulcers and points of cicatrization side by side. in tuberculosis nothing but progressive destruction.

PLATE XX.

Fig. 72.   Extensive destruction of the mandible.

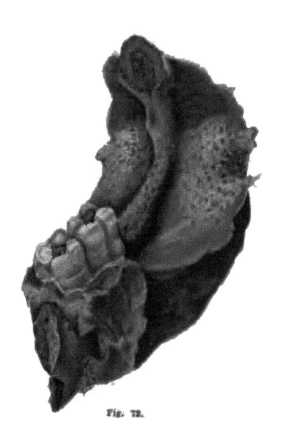

Fig. 72.

PLATE XX.

The presence of profuse granulations, unaccompanied by ulceration, speaks strongly for their lupoid character whether or not there is skin involvement. Extensive infiltration is likewise in favor of lupus.

Contrary to the commonly accepted assumption that the tuberculous cases occur most frequently in men, in contradistinction to lupus, I have been unable to find any striking dissimilarity in the two conditions. A large series of cases shows the following:

	Men	Women
Lupus	34.4%	65.6%
Tuberculosis	30.5%	69.2%

The age offers a better index: lupus occurs most frequently about the time of puberty and tuberculosis between the ages of twenty and fifty.

Caboche, who attempts to draw a sharp line between the lupic and tuberculous lesions, gives the following points upon which the differential diagnosis is to be based:

"1. We can surely list as pituitary lupus the cases of tuberculosis where there is remarked one or several of the following signs:"

"Mammillated infiltration of the mucosa, which I regard as the typical lesion of lupus."

"Perforation of the septal cartilage."

"Destruction of the alae nasi."

"Coexistence of other lupic lesions of the nose, cheek and face in general."

"Coexistence of other lupic lesions of the mucosa."

"Narinal atresia in tunnel form."

"2. We can almost, with certainty, include as lupus the cases where one of the following signs is shown:"

"Long duration of the affection."

"Frequent recrudescences in spite of methodical treatment."

"Lymphangitis of the lobule."

"The presence of vermicular cicatrices of the lobule or at the narinal orifices."

"The presence of 'eczema' of the nares, which, in several cases, seems to me to have been nothing else than vestibular lupus."

"These signs acquire the value of certainty if they coexist with one of the symptoms above mentioned."

"The absolute indolence of lupus contrasts with the pain, often sharp, of miliary tubercular ulcerations."

"I may add that the rarity or absence of bacilli upon histologic examination is also in favor of lupus."

Aside from syphilis and lupus, the only conditions capable of causing confusion are the new growths, either benign or malignant.

Certain cases of tuberculomata have some resemblance to simple mucous polypi, but the latter are generally multiple, have their attachment usually in the middle meatus or ethmoidal region and are more pedunculated, movable, compressible and transparent than the tuberculous growths.

The diagnostic features of the malignant growths are fully considered in the chapter on Diagnosis, Part I, and need not be here reiterated.

As a final diagnostic recourse we have the histologic demonstration of tuberculous tissue and the discovery of the bacillus in the secretions and scrapings.

As is the case with the larynx, anti-syphilitic treatment may cause temporary improvement of the tuberculous lesions, but this betterment is fleeting and at the end of two or three weeks all evidences of the improvement have usually disappeared.

PROGNOSIS.

Nasal tuberclosis, in itself and uncomplicated, is the least fatal form of phthisis and runs an exceedingly sluggish course. It occasions but little depression and malnutrition, and hence, unless it extends to the meninges or provokes constitutional tuberculosis, may endure for many years.

In some instances the disease has spread to the eye by way of the lachrimal duct, the cervical glands are often infected, and when the posterior part of the nose is diseased the process may extend to the nasopharynx.

The lymphatic glands become involved in a considerable number of cases, at least twenty-five per cent showing some enlargement. The cervical, submaxillary, sublingual and preauricular glands have all been involved, sometimes on one side only and occasionally on both sides.

Involvements of the tear-ducts have been especially considered by Caboche (*Ann. des Mal. de l'Oreille, du Lar., du Nez et du Phar.*, Sept., 1906).

He claims there is a form of vegetating nasal tuberculosis having its origin in the inferior meatus which rapidly invades the tear-ducts, constituting a nasolachrimal tuberculosis. It occurred in thirteen of twenty-four cases of nasal lupus.

The symptoms are nasal obstruction and epiphora. The objective symptoms consist of hypertrophy of the inferior turbinated body concealing fungous lesions of

the meatus, lachrimal fistula and cutaneous tuberculosis as an early sequel. In five out of nine cases reported by Kingsberg the disease extended from the
nose to the lachrimal duct and eye.

Each new focus means a corresponding decrease in
the chances of eventual arrest.

Even in the apparently primary cases, relapses
after the lesions are seemingly arrested or cured are
very common.

With the secondary lesions the prognosis depends
almost entirely upon the extent of involvement in the
other organs, the general nutrition, &c. It is as a rule
a late complication and therefore increases greatly
the gravity of the general prognosis. The local lesions
themselves seldom cicatrize unless seen and vigorously
treated during the stage of sharp circumscription.

The lupic cases are generally amenable to treatment
although they pursue a very protracted course.

TREATMENT.

The treatment of nasal tuberculosis should follow the
general lines laid down for the larynx. Where possible, the disease should be treated as a local tuberculosis and be thoroughly eradicated. Surgical treatment is always advisable provided the disease is local
and has resisted simple treatment; if it is a secondary
localization and the general prognosis is unfavorable,
no attempt at removal should be made unless the lesion
is both accessible and sharply circumscribed. If the
disease is not extensive it exerts but little influence
upon the constitutional condition, and an extensive

operation, even if it gave promise of completely curing the nose, would have a deletrious effect in general.

A. Onodi (*Deutsche med. Wochenschr.*, July 19, 1906) recommends for primary disease of the septum, of large extent, that the nasal cavity be opened in the median line with osteoplastic resection of the nasal bone and the frontal process of the superior maxillary, followed by complete resection of the involved portions of the septum.

As the process is practically painless we are seldom confronted with the alternative that so frequently presents in the larynx, and hence but two lines of treatment are to be considered: complete removal when the disease is circumscribed and the general disease amenable to treatment, and symptomatic management when the organic tuberculosis is advanced and the nasal lesion widespread. In the former case a complete cure may frequently be attained.

CHAPTER XVI.

THE NASOPHARYNX.

History.

The general recognition and study of tuberculous lesions of the nasopharynx is largely a development of the past decade, yet nearly thirty-five years have passed since the first authentic observations were recorded.

The pioneer work was done by Wendt, who in 1874 (*Krankheiten d. Nasenrachenhöhle u. d. Rachens. Ziemss, Handbuch, Bd.* VII, I.) brought the subject into prominence by his statement that tuberculous ulcers appear occasionally within the post-nasal space and that their point of election is the third tonsil, although the region about the orifices of the eustachian tubes is also occasionally invaded.

Little of additional value was adduced until six years later, when Barth and Zawerthal, in independent theses, drew attention anew to the subject.

The former (*De la Tuberculose du Pharynx et de l'angine tubercl.*) described three cases, in one of which, a lesion secondary to extensive ulceration of the posterior and lateral walls of the pharynx, there was deep ulceration and total destruction of the eustachian orifices.

Zawerthal (*Wien. Med. Presse,* 41-43, 1880) first advanced the fact of the occasional *primary* localization of the tuberculous process in the nasopharynx.

In the following year, 1881, E. Fränkel (*Anat. u. Klin. z. Lehre v. d. Erkrank. d. Nasenrachenraumes u. Gehörorganes b. Lungenschwinds., Zeitschr. f. Ohrenheilk.,* X, 2 *Heft*) published the results of fifty autopsies upon persons dead of consumption. In ten of these cases there was tuberculous ulceration of the postnasal space, generally of the tissues contiguous to the tubal apertures.

Not one case of acute miliary tuberculosis was included in this series.

Fränkel maintained that under certain conditions these ulcers might remain latent and be discovered only through anatomical examination, and that while they usually develop in patients with advanced pulmonary or other organic tuberculous disease, they occur rarely in individuals having but slight involvement. An extension of the process to the ear had not occurred in a single one of these patients.

Additional cases were now reported in quick succession, by Hinkel, Suchannek, Michelson, Northrup, and others.

In Hinkel's patient (Report of a case of Tubercular Ulceration of the Pharynx, Western New York Med. Press, May, 1886) there was ulceration of the nasal surface of the soft palate in association with extensive tuberculous disease of the larynx, tonsils and pharynx.

Suchannek (*Beitr. z. norm. u. path. Anat. d. Rachengewölbes, Ziegler's Beitr. z. Path, Anat.,* Bd. III, 1888) supported Fränkel's statement that ulcers of

the vault might remain a long time latent, and likewise advanced the fact that some apparently simple
erosions show tubercle bacilli upon microscopical examination.

In 1889, M. Hajek of Vienna (*D. Tuberc. d. Nasenschleimhaut, Klin. Rundschau., S.* 118) brought forward the first case of a tuberculous tumor in this locality. The growth was situated upon the upper surface of the soft palate and there was also tuberculous
ulceration of the nose, involving the cartilaginous septum. In this case the lesion was undoubtedly secondary to pulmonary consumption, there having been a
history of a previous hemorrhage.

Two years later Schnitzler (*Beitr. z. Kenntn. d. Tu-
berculinwirkung, Wein Klin. Wochenschr.*, 12, 1891)
placed on record a very unusual case of tumor formation resulting from the injection of tuberculin. This
patient, a man 31 years of age, had tuberculosis of the
lungs and larynx but the nasopharynx was apparently
unaffected, and yet, some days after the use of the
tuberculin, miliary tubercles appeared. The involvement of the nasopharynx followed a miliary outbreak
in the pharynx and this had been preceded for some
days by a similar eruption upon the epiglottis. At the
pharyngeal vault the nodules rapidly enlarged and
coalesced until a tumor of large size resulted. The
continued use of tuberculin, however, caused the
growth to break down and ulcerate, with eventual healing.

In regard to the frequency with which tuberculous
lesions of this region occur, the most valuable contri-
butions were made by Dmochowski (*Ueb. sec. Affect*

d. Nasenrachenhöhle b. Phthisikern., Ziegler's *Beitr. z. Path. Anat., Bd. XVI.*, 1894). He examined 64 consumptives, including eight cases of acute miliary tuberculosis, and found 21 with tuberculous invasion of the nasopharynx and in consequence of these findings reached the conclusion that secondary affections of the post-nasal tissues are very common, and that they are especially frequent in cases of acute miliary tuberculosis.

Habermann (cited by *Thost. Monatsschr. f. Ohrenheilk.*, 1896) met with two cases of ulceration in eight cases which he examined, but the great majority of the authorities, however, looked upon this case as a most uncommon manifestation of the disease.

Cases of tumors, in addition to those of Hajek and Schnitzler already cited, were recorded by Touton (*IV Congr. d. Deutschen Dermat. Ges.*, 1894); Koschier (*Ueb. Nasentuberculose. Wiener Klin. Wochenschr,* 36-42, 1895); Avellis (Cited by M. Schmidt) and others.

One of the earliest communications respecting the localization of the disease in the pharyngeal tonsil was made by Trautmann (*Anat. Pathol. u. Klin. Studien ueb. Hyperplasie d. Rachentonsille,* Berlin) in 1886. He declared that tuberculosis was nearly always the cause of adenoid growths, and in a later work (*Schwartze's Handbuch d. Ohrenheilk.*, Bd. II, S. 135, 1893) he maintained his former position, although admitting the general impossibility of demonstrating either giant cells or bacilli in the glandular tissues.

He based his conclusions on the well established fact that a large proportion of the children of consumptive parents have adenoid vegetations, and also upon the positive results of the tuberculin test in many instances.

In a large majority of the cases of pharyngeal tonsil hyperplasia, the injection of tuberculin produced some pyrexia with an increase in the local tumefaction. The continued use. of the tuberculin, however, led usually to the gradual retrogression of these symptoms, with eventual disappearance of the adenoids.

While few succeeding authors adopted the advanced stand taken by Trautmann, still the steadily increasing number of cases in which the tonsillar localization was proven, either with or without visible increase in size, directed attention to its possibility and caused painstaking examinations to be made in a large number of cases.

Few of the early examinations, however, revealed either giant cells or bacilli. Cornil (*Tuberculose larvée des trois amygdales, Ac. de med. de Paris*, 1895) made examinations of 70 hypertrophied tonsils without finding bacilli in a single case and giant cells only four times. Of ten specimens examined by Pilliet (*Soc. Anatom.*, March 25, 1892), three contained giant cells but bacilli were totally lacking.

The majority of the investigators, including Seifert, Kahn, Châtelier, Luc, and Dubief, were unable to find any evidences of tubercle formation in extirpated tonsils, but it is perhaps possible that the negative results depended upon the fact that the sections did not pass through the affected areas and that only a few sections were made, for it is now a well known fact that the process is always localized in certain areas and is never diffused throughout the entire gland. A localized involvement may, therefore, be easily overlooked.

On the other hand, a number of positive results were soon recorded. Both bacilli and giant cells were found in the adenoid tissue by Lermoyez; in 32 cases, offering no macroscopic evidences of phthisis, he found tubercles in two. In several additional cases pulmonary tuberculosis developed upon the removal of the growths.

So many cases of this kind, i. e., instances of disseminated tuberculous infections following the removal of hyperplastic pharyngeal tonsils, have now been assembled, in addition to those in which microscopic evidences of the disease have been found, that a doubt can no longer exist that the condition is comparatively frequent and that this lymphatic tissue is a not uncommon portal through which the bacilli gain entrance into the body.

ETIOLOGY.

Post-nasal tuberculosis is usually secondary to far advanced disease of other organs but apparently primary cases, particularly of the tonsil, have been recorded in a considerable number of instances.

As to the frequency of tuberculous involvements of the nasopharynx it is almost impossible to quote figures of definite worth, because of the fact that in the majority of instances there are no macroscopical alterations, and deductions must therefore be drawn almost entirely from microscopical examination of excised tonsils and animal inoculations.

From the following tables a fairly clear idea may be had, however, of the frequency of the various types:

Of these cases the diagnosis in seven (those of Cornil and Pilliet) was based upon the presence of giant cells alone, no bacilli having been found.

A number of other cases have been uncovered by means of inoculation tests upon guinea pigs.

C

Author.	Inoculation Tests.	Tuberculosis.
Lewin	100	10
Baup	45	1
Dieulafog	35	7
Lartigan & Nicoll	75	12
Wright	12	0
Total	267	30

In a total of 1837 cases there were 115 of nasopharyngeal tuberculosis, or 6.2 per cent.

Of these cases 1026 were consumptives, and of them 54, or 5.2 per cent, had ulcerative lesions that were macroscopically recognizable.

The remaining 811 cases, individuals apparently free from tuberculosis, from whom the adenoid tissue was removed and examined, showed tuberculosis in 61, or 7.5 per cent.

When there is advanced disease of the lungs, however, and particularly when complicated by laryngeal involvement, the percentage of tonsillar involvements is greatly increased; thus in 136 such cases the tonsils were tuberculous in 94, or 68 per cent.

The large majority of the ulcerative lesions are secondary in nature but a few of apparently primary origin have been noted, especially by Dmochowski, who in three cases believed the tonsillar lesion to have been the cause of acute miliary tuberculosis.

Hurd (*Laryngoscope*, July, 1907) reported an interesting case of an apparently primary tuberculous growth of the nasopharynx that occupied the vault and posterior wall. The growth was slightly nodular and covered by a normal appearing mucous membrane.

The report of the pathologist, Dr. Jonathan Wright, was as follows: "Microscopic examination of a piece removed by forceps shows that in mounting the hardened specimen crumbled from the hardening process. Many of the fragments show very plainly perfectly typical tubercle. Centres of tubercle granulum or necrobiosis are surrounded by a rim of new connective tissue in attempts at repair. In a few of these areas may be seen a typical Langerhans giant cell. Some of the round cell tissue apparently at a distance from the tubercles is altered somewhat by chronic inflammation and contains no lymph nodes. The tubercular tissue, or rather the tubercle granula, are not immediately under the epithelium which is fairly normal columnar, but separated from it by a rim of lymph cells. This is the second case only which I have seen in which there were multiple tubercles in a posterior lymphoid hypertrophy, the other having been from the service of Dr. Chappell and reported by me with a color plate in the New York Medical Journal, Sept. 26, 1896. Perhaps, owing to the scantiness of the lymphoid tissue, there being no nodes, it is not accurate to call this tubercle of the adenoid, but of the nasopharynx.''

"A search of 10 sections failed to reveal any tubercle bacilli.''

"March 15, 1906. Two guinea pigs inoculated.''

"June 6th, 1906. One of the guinea pigs inoculated two months before with pieces of the growth removed from the naso-pharynx beneath the skin of abdomen showed enlarged inguinal glands. The other guinea pig showed beginning round celled infiltration (presumably tuberculosis) of the smaller bronchi.''

SOURCE OF INFECTION.

The chief factor in etiology consists in the peculiar anatomical conformation of the parts. We have to deal with a sort of sac or pouch, blind upon its superior and posterior aspects, but communicating from its anterior surface with the nose, and inferiorly with the pharynx and mouth and through these latter channels with the larynx and lungs.

The space is therefore open to infection from two sides: from the nose by inhalation or extension by contiguity, and from the lower segments of the respiratory tract by direct transference of bacilli in sputum and vomitus, as well as by direct spread. The conformation of the remaining parts, the blind surface of the pouch, favors the indefinite retention and growth of all germs so deposited.

At the upper end of the sac, the point where the inspired air current strikes with greatest force and therefore where the largest deposit of germs occurs, the mucosa is thrown into a number of uneven folds and furrows by a considerable collection of lymphatic tissue, the so-called Luschka's, or third tonsil. Even in its normal state this gland offers a favorable culture field by reason of its uneven surface and deep crypts, within which the epithelial lining is often desquamated. This nidus is rendered still more fertile, however, by reason of the fact that it is both inflamed and enlarged in the great majority of all consumptives. In children under the age of puberty some enlargement of the tonsil, and therefore an increase in the depth of the crypts, is almost always present, and in many cases it is of a degree sufficient to give rise to the condition recognized as adenoids.

Both of these conditions, glandular hypertrophy and simple inflammation or catarrh, strongly favor infection, because the consequent narrowing of the respiratory channel causes the air to impinge with unnatural force against the damaged tissue, the crypts form a barrier to the expulsion of the bacilli thus deposited, and their penetration into the deeper structures is facilitated by the numerous erosions existent and by the frequent replacement of the normal ciliated epithelium by one of a squamous type. As has been shown to be the case with the larynx, some antecedent weakening of the tissues is almost invariably necessary to the development of the tubercle bacilli; in other words, a point of *locus minoris resistentia* must have been created and this favorable soil is produced by both of these above considered conditions.

That inhalation infection does not occur with even greater frequency is due to the arrest of the majority of all foreign bodies in the anterior chambers of the nose. The effectiveness of the nasal passages as a filter has been proven by various experiments, only a few of which need be here cited:

Of 29 apparently normal men examined by Strauss, 9 had tubercle bacilli in the nasal secretions.

Hildebrandt (*Exper. Unters. über d. Eindringen pathogener Mikroorganismen v. d. Luftwegen, u. d. Lunge aus. Ziegler's Beitr. z. path. Anat., Bd.* II, 1888) subjected rabbits to the nasal inhalation of *Aspergillus Fumigatus* without the production of any pulmonary changes, but when the inhalations were given through a tracheal cannula the characteristic hepatization readily occurred.

In The Medical Record of August 25, 1900, W. Noble Jones reported the results of his experiments in injecting guinea pigs with the nasal secretions of average healthy persons not unduly associated with consumptives, in which he had a positive result in 10.3 per cent of the cases. (See Page 266).

Those organisms that succeed in passing through the nose are deposited, as a rule, in the region between the roof of the nose and the posterior wall, the area occupied by Luschka's gland and where the conditions are most favorable for their development.

There are several additional factors, however, which under normal conditions militate strongly against infection. In the first place the epithelium is of the ciliated variety and tends to expel all foreign bodies there deposited; *secondly*, there is a film of tenacious mucus such as exists in the nose that prevents their deposit or long retention, and *thirdly*, the tubercle bacillus requires a considerable period of time in which to develop and produce pathologic changes in the tissues.

Under two conditions, however, these defenses may prove inadequate: *First*, when points of *locus minoris resistentiae* exist, and *second*, when large numbers of tubercle bacilli are simultaneously introduced.

We have seen that adenoid vegetations act as a strong predisposing moment and retro-nasal catarrh is almost equally potent. This has been clearly shown by Freudenthal (*Kleinere Beitr. z. Aet. d. Lungentuberculose, Arch. f. Laryng., Bd. V*, 1896) in his examinations of the post-nasal secretions of 133 patients of the Montefiore Home who had no symptoms referable to the nose or throat.

Of these patients 52 were tuberculous and 81 non-tuberculous. Of the 52 with consumption, 21 had nasopharyngeal catarrh, and of the 81 non-tubercluous, 34.

Tubercle bacilli were found in the secretions of 24 of the cases of tuberculosis and in nine of those not suffering from the disease. Certain of the non-tuberculous cases that had bacilli in the secretions developed tuberculosis later, strong presumptive evidence that the disease had its primary localization in the naso-pharynx.

Atrophic rhinitis must be looked upon as an import-ant predisposing factor in some cases. In this disease the physiologic functions of the nose, as a filterer and moistener of the inspired air, are almost entirely de-stroyed, for in place of the normal convolutions the passages are wide and straight and the mucosa is more or less completely deprived of its normal secre-tions and cilia.

As a result, the majority of the foreign bodies that are drawn into the nose, instead of being arrested near the introitus pass through and are deposited in the nasopharynx, and as there is always an accompanying nasopharyngitis in this condition, the bacilli find a favorable field for development.

While inhalation undoubtedly plays the most import-ant role in the etiology of post-nasal tuberculosis, the disease in some instances is due to lymphatic and blood transmission, in others to infection from the lower seg-ments of the respiratory tract. In the act of coughing, particles of infected sputum may be thrown into the nasopharynx and vomiting sometimes results in con-siderable quantities of food being forced up behind the palate, while in the majority of cases of laryngeal tu-berculosis accompanied by dysphagia and odynopha-gia, some regurgitation of food, both liquid and solid, accompanies almost every effort at deglutition.

The imperfect apposition of the palate to the poste-rior wall, through which this entrance of food and sputum into the post-nasal space is made possible, is due to one of two causes: in coughing incomplete clos-

PLATE XXI.

Fig. 73. Tuberculosis of the pharyngeal tonsil, with sinus leading to necrotic bone.

PLATE XXI.

Fic. 73. Tuberculosis of the pharyngeal tonsil.

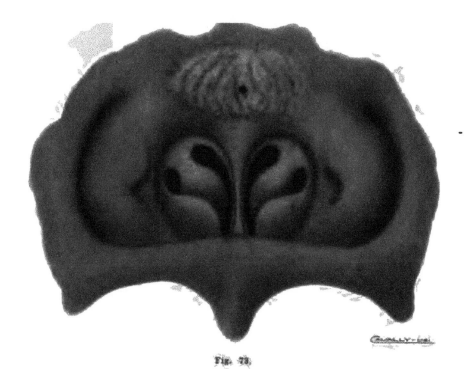

Fig. 78.

PLATE

ure may result from attempts at suppression through keeping the mouth tightly closed, a common practice with consumptives when in the presence of strangers or at the table; an additional cause is undoubtedly to be found in that tumefaction of the parts which is a not uncommon accompaniment of laryngeal tuberculosis.

These factors explain why infections in the region of the pharyngeal tonsil occur chiefly during the late stages of phthisis pulmonalis.

An active but rather rare cause in advanced cases is direct extension of the process from neighboring foci, i. e., in the nose, sinuses, pharynx, buccal cavity, &c.

Just what role the primary infections of the nasopharyngeal lymphatic tissue play in the development of tuberculosis of other organs cannot be definitely determined, but it can no longer be doubted that they are of great etiologic moment.

In a not inconsiderable number of primary pharyngeal tonsil infections an acute miliary tuberculosis of the lungs has been super-added, and the majority of cases of cervical lymphadenitis may be traced to disease of the pharyngeal and faucial tonsils. Both pulmonary and laryngeal foci have oftimes resulted, according to many authorities, from preceding disease of the cervical glands.

On the other hand, the process may remain latent for a long time or even be permanently arrested and leave no trace of its previous existence.

The question is not entirely academic for it has a strong bearing upon the problem of operative intervention; whether the infective focus should be radically extirpated to prevent further dissemination, or whether, on the other hand, such procedures favor extension to new organs or ulceration at the point of excision.

This point has not been definitely settled but it appears reasonable to conclude that excision, as with tuberculous processes of other organs that are purely local, will afford the best chance of permanent arrest.

When such enlargements exist, aside from their baneful effects upon the general nutrition which would favor the development of tuberculosis in those otherwise predisposed, there is constant danger of acute inflammatory processes supervening, which are even more liable to cause dissemination than the traumatism arising from a clean and rapidly healing wound.

That delayed healing may occasionally result in these cases, however, has been shown by Hessler (*Ueb. d. Operat. d. aden. Vegetat. m. d. neuen Schütz'schen Pharyngotonsillstom., Münch. med. Wochenschr.. 29, 1895*). He operated one child and resolution was normal, but in her sister healing was greatly delayed; there was great swelling of the cervical glands, profuse secretions, fever and general prostration that lasted for weeks. It only subsided when the child was removed to a more favorable climate. There was tuberculosis in the family and several had died of it, and this child, in physical characteristics, resembled these members.

Extension may likewise occur even when the gland has not been subject to traumatism, hence the existence of such an area is a constant menace for not alone are there possibilities of pulmonary and glandular infections, but of aural involvements and of extension to the retropharyngeal glands and meninges as well.

OBJECTIVE SYMPTOMS.

Three forms of nasopharyngeal tuberculosis are clinically recognizable:

1. Involvement of the adenoid tissue.
2. Ulceration.
3. Tumors.

1. *The Pharyngeal Tonsil.* The frequency and etiologic factors concerning tuberculosis of the lymphatic glands of the vault have already been considered, so there remain for discussion only the clinical and diagnostic features.

Considerable enlargement, when occurring in individuals with well marked involvement of the lungs or other organs, may safely be looked upon as tuberculous for the vast majority of such cases have been proven to be so, but in the absence of other signs of the disease, histologic examination of the excised tissue or animal inoculations can alone determine whether the hyperplasia is due to simple inflammatory changes or to a latent tuberculous focus.

There may be widespread tuberculous involvement without macroscopic alterations and this is indeed the usual condition, as has been shown in considering the etiology of the laryngeal lesions.

Seifert (*Heymann's Handbuch der Laryngologie und Rhinologie*, p. 719), in determining the probability of an hypertrophy being due to tuberculosis, directs attention to the following points:

(1). History, heredity, &c.

(2). Existence of other scrofulo-tuberculous signs in the skin or glands.

(3). Severe disturbances of nutrition not in har-
mony with the usual picture of adenoids.

Several investigators claim that tuberculosis is the
almost invariable cause of glandular overgrowth, but
this advanced hypothesis is not substantiated by pathologic study, which shows only an approximate five
per cent in which indisputable evidences of tuberculosis have been found.

On the other hand it cannot be gainsaid that the hypertrophies occur most frequently in the children of
tuberculous parents or of families some members of
which have the disease, and there is usually simultaneous enlargement of other lymphatic tissues, i. e., the
faucial tonsils, lingual and cervical glands.

Aside from the hyperplasia there are no symptoms
evoked, either local or constitutional, through which a
differential diagnosis is made possible.

It is well to reiterate at this point that latent tuberculosis of this tissue may exist without any increase in
size, and even in glands that have become atrophic.

Whether the hypertrophy usually depends upon the
bacillary infection or whether there is generally a
preceding enlargement upon which the tuberculous process is grafted, is disputed, but we can state quite pos-
itively that both theories are tenable. It has been shown
that the disease is sometimes found in normal sized
tonsils and even in those which have undergone atrophy, and certain histological and clinical considerations point to the assumption that the hypertrophy usually precedes the bacillary infection.

The tuberculosis is limited to the lymphoid tissue and
does not involve the submucosa, and the bacilli are met

PLATE XXII.

Fig. 74. Ulceration of the nasal surface of the soft palate
and uvula, secondary to advanced disease of the
pharynx.

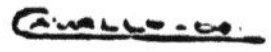

Fig. 74.

PLATE

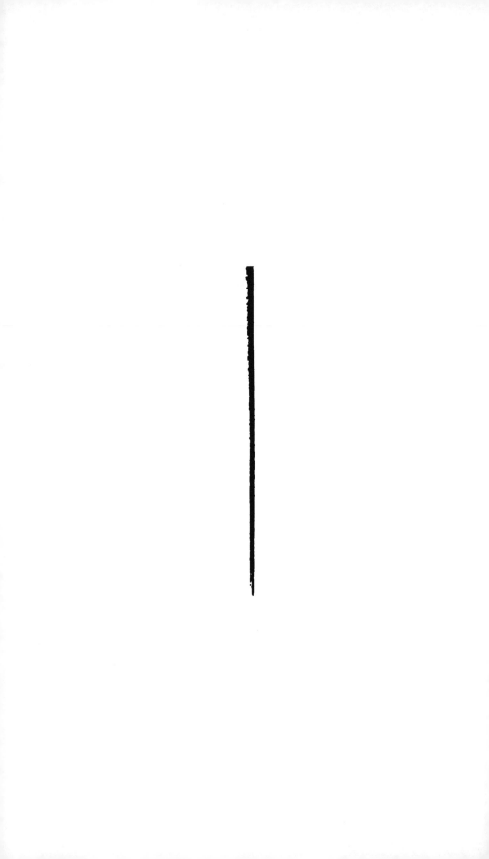

with only in the affected areas and never in the healthy
lymph follicles or upon the epithelium.

The process is not a diffuse one but is circumscribed
to certain segments; it may involve an entire lobe of the
gland or only certain portions of it, while the neighboring lobes remain entirely normal.

If the hyperplasia invariably depended upon bacillary infection, it would be rational to conclude that occasionally the disease would be found more or less diffused throughout the entire gland, in place of the constant limitation to circumscribed segments and tissues.

Certain clinical phenomena uphold this idea, i. e.,
the infection of an already existing hyperplasia; recurrences after extirpation are exceedingly uncommon,
transmission to other organs is rare and the process
is usually completely checked.

That the hyperplasia does in certain instances depend entirely upon the tuberculous infection cannot be
gain-said any more than the contrary view, but all considerations point to the probability that there is in the
majority of cases a primary enlargement.

In determining whether or not a latent lesion is present in the nasopharynx, the opthalmo-reaction of Cal-
mette may prove of some service. The injection into
the eye of a solution of dry tuberculin, precipitated by
alcohol at 95 degrees, in distilled and sterilized water,
usually produces a congestion of the tarsal conjunctiva within three to five hours, although it may be delayed 24 or even 48 hours, provided the body conceals
a tuberculous lesion. The membrane becomes a bright
red in color and there is more or less edema and moderate lachrimation.

di. Med., Turin, Nov., 1907), there resulted an increased activity in the lungs and glands, with general phenomena.

Lewin (*Archiv. für Rhinol. u. Laryngol., Berlin*, B. 9, H. 3) bases the following conclusions upon the results of an examination of 200 subjects:

"(1). According to our investigations, hyperplastic pharyngeal tonsils conceal tuberculous lesions in about 5 per cent of the cases.

"(2). The tuberculosis is present in the so-called tumor form, it is characterized by the absence of surface indications of its presence—latent tuberculosis of the tonsils.

"(3). This 'latent' tuberculosis may apparently be

the first and indeed the only localization of the disease in the individual.

"(4). It is generally, however, associated with other tuberculous processes, generally of the lungs, which may, however, not have developed at the time the tonsil was operated upon.

"(5). It is a comparatively frequent condition among those suffering from tuberculosis of the lungs.

"(6). It is found in the normal sized tonsil as well as in the hyperplastic. Whether it may cause hyperplasia by the development of some toxin is doubtful. It can, however, retard the normal involution of the tonsil.

"(7). Its part in the etiology of hypertrophy of the pharyngeal tonsil is unimportant.

"(8). By removal of the tonsil the disease may be removed, even though tuberculosis of the lungs be present."

2. *The Ulcer.* Tuberculous ulceration in the nasopharynx may occur either as a primary or secondary manifestation of the disease, but the latter represents the by far more common type although a considerable number of apparently primary cases are recorded.

The condition is seldom recognized clinically owing to the fact that systematic examinations are rarely made in advanced cases of phthisis unless severe subjective throat symptoms are evoked, but in post-mortems upon people dead of consumption it is found in a not inconsiderable percentage of the cases.

This discrepancy has already been shown; ulcers were found in ten of 50 consumptives examined post-mortem (20 per cent), while in 904 living cases of local despite painstaking rhinoscopic and post-rhinoscopic examination of every consumptive, and Schmidt has had the same experience. .

The ulcer in this space has the same characteristics as tuberculous ulcers of other mucous membranes and demands no separate description. Its chief point of difference consists in its tendency to spread towards the depths and involve the deeper structures more rapidly and constantly than does its laryngeal prototype. (Plate XXI, Fig. 73.)

The lymphatic tissue usually melts away with surprising rapidity, as is seen in cases where the faucial tonsils are secondarily involved. The base is nearly always uneven and covered by profuse granulations and tenacious muco-purulent secretions, and the pa-

PLATE XXIII.

Fig. 75. Tuberculosis limited to the posterior lip of the Eustachian tube and Rosenmueller's fossa.

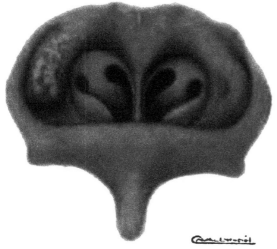

Fig. 73.

PLATE XXIII.

thognomonic miliary tubercles are usually to be seen
about the ulcers and in the adjacent membranes.

The process is occasionally localized upon the upper
surface of the soft palate, and I have seen one case in
which the ulcers were limited to Rosenmüller's fossa
and the posterior lip of the tube. (Figs. 74 and 75,
Plates 22 and 23.)

The prognosis is generally unfavorable. in that the
lesion nearly always occurs late in the course of pulmonary and laryngeal tuberculosis; in such instances
symptomatic treatment is alone justifiable. Some of
the cases, however, run a typically latent course. If,
on the other hand, the nasopharyngeal disease is primary or an accompaniment of only moderate disease
elsewhere, complete extirpation may produce an enduring cure.

Both the local and constitutional treatment is identical with that outlined for the larynx.

3. *The Tumor.* That the tuberculous tumor of the
nasopharynx may be the sole apparent localization of
the disease in the individual, as has already been shown
to be the case with tuberculomata of the larynx and
nose, is demonstrated by a case studied by Koschier
(*Ueb. Nasentuberculose, Wien Klin. Wochenschr.,*
36-42, 1895).

In this patient the entire post-nasal space was occupied by a smooth, pale red tumor that was divided
by sulci into numerous lobules. There was no ulceration of the surface, and microscopic examination
proved the growth to be tuberculous although at no
time was there any evidence of pulmonary or laryngeal
disease.

be considered in the same light as other new growths and complete removal is to be practiced in every case, even when there is advancd disease of the lungs or other organs. Recurrences have been noted but the prognosis is generally favorable.

CHAPTER XVII.

THE PHARYNX.

History.

No section of the respiratory tract succumbs so rapidly to the ravages of tuberculosis when a focus is once established, nor leads to such hopeless suffering, as the pharynx.

The infections occur in such a manner that all preventive measures are entirely gratuitous and since curative and even palliative treatment, when the disease has once gained headway, is absolutely ineffective in the vast majority of cases, a study of the disease can lead to little of practical value beyond the possibility of establishing an early diagnosis.

Primary disease of the tonsils, on the other hand, since it is generally of the so-called latent type, is amendable to surgical treatment, and hence it is extremely important that the physician should never lose sight of the fact that these organs are infected in a considerable percentage of all cases of hyperplasia, and even in some that have undergone atrophy, and that they play a most important role in the dissemination of the disease to other structures.

While this latter form is of comparatively recent recognition, dating from the classical paper by Dieulafoy, read in 1895 before the Paris Academy of Medicine, the ulcerative involvements of the pharynx were well described as far back as 1871. In this year Isambert first brought the subject into prominence by his paper entitled, "*De la tubercul. miliaire aigue pharyngo-laryngée.*"

This communication was followed by two others, the one, "*Nouv. faits de tuberculose miliaire de la gorge,*" published in 1876, and the other, "*Confér. clin. s. l. mal. du larynx,*" in the following year. In this latter paper he described an apparently primary case that occurred in a boy four and a half years of age.

Until this time the condition had been practically neglected, as is shown by Wendt (Ziemssen's *Handbuch,* 1874) in his statement, "Concerning the occurrence of tubercles in the throat, little is known."

Aside from Isambert, the most valuable contribution to the literature of this period was made by B. Fränkel, in 1876 (*Ueb. d. Miliartuberculose d. Pharynx, Berliner Klin. Wochenschr.*)

In this thesis he said that only one case of tuberculous ulceration of the pharynx had been found in 150 consumptive cadavers examined at the Berlin Pathological Institute, and also declared that the majority of the cases occur during childhood and adolescence.

Several years before this, Navratil (*Laryn. Beitr.,* Leipzig, 1871) had reported seeing 246 cases of ulceration of the larynx and pharynx. Of these, 162 were tuberculous, 44 syphilitic, and 30 scrofulous, and in 20 of the tuberculous patients there was ulceration of the pharynx. Whether or not these were all true tuberculous ulcerations cannot now be determined.

Barth (*De la tuberculose du pharynx*), in 1880, assembled 35 cases, of which two were individuals over 60 years of age. Birch-Hirschfeld (*Lehrbuch d. path. Anat.*, Leipzig, 1877) maintained that while tuberculous ulceration of the pharynx might occur as a primary condition, it is almost invariably a consequence of preceding disease of other organs, and Küssner (*Ueb. prim. Tuberc. d. Gaumen, Deutsche med. Wochenschr.*, 1881) reported five primary cases, all occuring in men between the years of 34 and 56.

Guttmann (*Tuberkelbacillen in tuberc. Geschwüren d. weichen Gaumens, Deutsche med. Wochenschr.*, 21, 1883) held that a primary localization of the disease in the pharynx never occurs.

Tuberculosis of the tonsils, in patients suffering from phthisis pulmonalis, in which the lesions were scarcely noticeable to the naked eye and unattended by subjective symptoms, was described by Cornil and Weigert as early as 1884. These observations may have been made upon cases which would to-day be considered "latent."

In the same year Strassmann (*Ueb. Tubercul. d. Tonsillen, Virch. Arch., Bd.* XCVI, 1884) examined 21 tonsils taken from subjects of tuberculosis and found tuberculous involvement in 15.

The occurrence of miliary tubercles of the tonsils during the course of general miliary tuberculosis was described by Cornil and Ranvier during this same period (*Man. d'histologie Path.*, 2 Edition, 1884).

Lublinski, 1887, (*Tuberc. d. Tonsillen, Monatschr, f. Ohrenheilk.*) observed two cases of tonsillar tuberculosis that were secondary to disease of both the lungs and larynx, while several observers, among whom may be mentioned Abraham, Franks, and L. Browne, brought forward cases of tonsillar disease that were apparently of a primary nature.

The first of these (Tubercle of the Tonsil, Dublin Journal of Medicial Science, Oct., 1885) demonstrated the presence of beginning caseation, with extensive tubercle formation, in the tonsil of a woman otherwise normal.

Schlenker (*Unters. über d. Entstehung d. Tuberc. d. Halslymphdrüsen, bes, ueber ihre Bezieh. z. Tubercul. d. Tonsillen*, Virch. Arch. Nr. 134, 1893) examined 24 cadavers in order to establish the relationship between tonsillar, cervical-glandular and pulmonary tuberculosis, and concluded that: "The cervical ganglia receive their infection from the tonsils, and that the latter receive their own from the lungs by means of the sputa."

This view was upheld by Krückmann (*Ueb. d. Bezieh. d. Tuberculose. d. Halslymphdrüsen su. d. Tonsillen*, Virch. Arch., Bd. CXX & CVIII, 1894) who observed tonsil tuberculosis in all of his 12 cases of cervical adenitis.

In the following year came the epoch-making communication of Dieulafoy, in which, for the first time, was strikingly advanced the theory of a latent tonsillar disease not provocative of any subjective or objective macroscopic symptoms.

His experiments were carried out by means of tonsil and adenoid injections into the abdomens of guinea pigs, which were then examined for signs of the disease.

Sixty-one tonsil inoculations were made, with the following results: 6 of the pigs died with evidence of tuberculosis at the point of inoculation and of general tuberculosis; 2 showed pulmonary without local tuberculosis; 4 had general sepsis and in 49 there was no apparent cause for death. 35 adenoid inoculations were made, and of these animals 3 died from both a local and pulmonary infection; 4 of pulmonary without local disease; 3 of sepsis and 25 without any demonstrable lesions.

From these results, which have been vigorously attacked, the theory of the frequent existence of a latent tuberculous lesion of the tonsils was evolved, and this assumption has been so many times substantiated by later and less impeachable experiments and clinical observations, that the doctrine has now gained almost universal and unquestioned acceptance.

ETIOLOGY.

Many of the etiologic factors in connection with pharyngeal tuberculosis have been considered in studying the larynx, nasopharynx and nose, hence only those phases of the subject that are of especial importance or that have not been previously considered, will be taken up.

Six channels of infection are recognized: (1) inhalation; (2) blood; (3) lymphatic vessels; (4) sputum; (5) ingesta; (6) direct extension from contiguous foci.

In the vast majority of all cases the pharyngeal involvement is secondary to more or less advanced disease of other structures, so in these instances we have to consider only four of these six possible routes: sputum, lymph, blood, and direct extension.

In the primary cases infection occurs through the air, food or drink.

Frequency: Pharyngeal tuberculosis is a relatively rare disease as can be seen from the following table:

	Inoculation Tests	*
		1
Lartigan & Nicoll................	75	12
Total	267	

Observer	nsump	Pharyngeal Cases
Heintz	1226	11
Willigk	*1307	1
Böcher.....................	2950	12
Fränkel.....................	*150	1
Lublinski	1600	5
Kidd	*500	7
Phipps Institute	†618	3
Walsham	*200	1
Levy	*500	67
Agnes Memorial Sanatorium.......	†638	1
Author	‡904	39
	10623	151=1.47%

† Consumptives.
‡ Laryngeal Cases.
* Autopsies.

Delavan (New York Med. Journ., May 14, 1887) in 100 cases of local tuberculosis, found the various structures affected as follows:

Pharynx 24
Tongue 37
Cheeks 22
Uvula 8
Nose 5
Tonsils 4

Guttmann places the proportion of pharyngeal cases in consumptives at 1 per cent, and Levy at 1 1-2 per cent, both of which correspond closely to the 1.47 per cent of the above table.

Rosenberg (*Quelques remarq. s. l. tuberc. laryngée, Rev. de lar.* 22, 1895) saw only 22 cases of pharyngeal tuberculosis in 22,000 patients with throat disease, three of which were apparently primary.

Considering the relative infrequency of infection and its exposed position, it must be granted that the pharynx has in itself or its secretions some property that is extremely antagonistic to the deposit or growth of the tubercle bacillus.

This theory of an active immunity holds whether the majority of infections are considered as endogenous or exogenous.

If the sputum constitutes the vehicle through which invasion occurs, why is it that the pharynx is so much less frequently affected than the larynx? The parts of the larynx that are covered by squamous epithelium are especially open to attack and yet corresponding parts of the pharynx, the lower posterior and lateral walls, where the sputum is much longer retained than in the larynx from whence it is soon removed by coughing, are only very rarely effected.

We are equally at a loss, on the other hand, if the infections are ascribed to blood and lymphatic transmission, for the pharynx is richly supplied with both blood and lymph vessels.

It has been abundantly proven that the tubercle bacilli penetrate normal intact epithelial surfaces and gland ducts, and yet, while the faucial, pharyngeal and lingual tonsils, and the bronchial glands are frequently primarily attacked, the posterior wall is rarely invaded in this way,—infection, when it does occur, being almost always consequent upon preceding disease of other organs.

To what factors, then, may this immunity be ascribed?

By some observers it has been claimed that the frequent passage of food, both solid and liquid, through keeping the pharyngeal wall in a state of almost constant excitation, prevents the lodgement and long retention of the bacilli at any one point, but this theory does not do away with the fact that during the hours of rest the throat is bathed almost continuously with infected pus and is left undisturbed. This explanation of the pharyngeal immunity has been subscribed to by both Schech (*Krankheiten der Mundhöhle*, p. 219) and Cornet (Tuberculosis, p. 126). The latter says:

"The inferior portion of the posterior wall of the pharynx, with its smooth surface and its rich secretion of mucus, does not afford conditions favorable to the growth of the tubercle bacillus, just as a much-trodden pathway through a meadow does not permit of the growth of grass, notwithstanding that the soil itself is in proper condition. For here, too, there is an incessant to-and-fro motion, food and drink passing downward, mucus travelling upward, so that the bacillus is denied the chance to gain a firm hold."

Walsham (Channels of Infection in Tuberculosis, p. 64-65) ascribes the immunity to the character of the normal secretions poured into the pharynx and to the normal resistance of the mucosa itself. He says:

"I think that in cases of tuberculosis of the pharynx we must assume some alteration in the secretions poured into the pharynx by the surrounding glands, or some alteration in the mucous membranes. A mere loss of its epithelial lining is not perhaps necessary for the penetration of the bacillus, because we now know that the bacillus can penetrate normal epithelium.

"Dr. Vincent Harris has shown that the salivary glands (the glands examined were the parotid and sub-maxillary) undergo marked histological changes in tuberculosis. Now although tubercle of the salivary glands is almost unknown, nevertheless in many cases of the disease they undergo a distinct histological change. Dr. Harris says: 'Having from a number of cases demonstrated the occasional deficiency in the amount of diastatic ferment of the saliva (ptyalin) of phthisical patients in a late stage of the disease, I undertook the examination of the salivary glands of such cases obtained from the post-mortem room, with the view of finding out whether the condition of the secreting tissue might not account for such deficiency. The examination of a few cases suggested a probable explanation of the abnormal secretion, namely, that fibrosis, sometimes sufficiently marked to be evident to the unaided eye, was not infrequently present.'

"I have seen this condition of fibrosis also in the tonsils in some cases of pulmonary tubercle.

"I think we may sum up by saying that, owing to some lesion of the pharyngeal wall or to alteration of the secretions poured into the pharynx, tuberculosis of this part of the alimentary tract may result."

When the defenses, whatever they may be, are weakened, infection occurs and probably in nearly all cases from sputal contact. It may very rarely be primary, or it may occur in the form of a miliary outbreak, either isolated or as part of a general miliary tuberculosis; in this type infection of course occurs through the blood.

. The failure of frequent lymphatic transmission may, perhaps, be ascribed to the poor anastomosis between the external and internal lymphatics. The infrequency of lymphatic spread from the larynx does not in any way militate against the theory of lymphatic infection of the larynx from the lungs, for, as pointed out by Friedrich, it is well known that in other laryngeal diseases, notably carcinoma, enlargement of the glands and extension to surrounding structures occur only in the later stages of the disease. This unique position of the laryngeal lymphatic system may account for the tendency of the disease to remain localized in the larynx.

Although the process in the preponderating majority of all cases is a secondary one, there are a few recorded instances in which it appeared to be the primary focus and in such instances infection must be accredited to the inspired air or to infected food.

The possibility of infected food causing tuberculosis of the tonsils has been shown by Orth and Baumgarten (Orth: *Exper. Unters. über die Fütterungstuberc.*, Virchow's Archives, Vol. LXVI). They fed animals with tuberculous tissue, and after a short time had elapsed always found tuberculosis of the cervical and bronchial glands, and later of the mesenteric glands, with demonstrable intestinal lesions.

Apparently primary cases have been recorded by Isambert; Pluder (1 case); Schleicher (1); Küssner (5 cases); Uckermann (1); Heymann (1); Wróblewski (1); Heller (1); Fränkel (1); Küer (1); Delavan (1); Crossfield (1); Clarke (1); Rosenberg (3); Roth (1); Seifert (2); and others.

Clarke's case concerned a boy eighteen years of age who had widespread lesions of the mouth and almost total destruction of the soft palate. The lungs, on post-mortem examination, were found to be absolutely normal.

The case reported by Isambert is not conclusive as the child had suffered from scrofula and obstinate rhinitis.

Willis, in a paper read before the American Academy of Ophthalmology and Oto-Laryngology, in 1907, referred to two cases of primary tuberculosis of the uvula, one a personal case, the other a patient seen by J. Braden Kyle. Willis's case, two years before the palatal tuberculosis was recognized, had been operated for a rectal fistula, and at that time an "ulcerated growth was found in the rectum, "which did not heal kindly." No autopsy was held.

In addition to these channels, i. e., food, air, sputum, blood and lymph, we have certain instances in which the disease has reached the pharynx by direct extension from the neighboring tissues.

A case of direct spread from the larynx is described by Rey (*Cas de phthisie laryngée avec. granulat. et ulcérat. tubercul. du pharynx et perforations de la paroi laryngo-pharyngienne, Progrès Méd.*, 18, 1885).

This patient, a man of 40 years, had necrosis of the posterior part of the cricoid cartilage, and from this focus the process spread to the pharynx.

V. Jaruntowski (*Z. Aetiol. d. tubercul. Affectionen
d. Mundhöhle, Münch. med. Wochenschr.*, 18, 1895)
described a case in which the disease reached the anterior pillar of the tonsil from a lesion of the cheek.

According to Löri (*D. durch, anderw. Erkrank. bed.
Veränderung d. Rachens. d. Kehlkopfes u. d. Luftrö
hre* 1885) there are sometimes found, in cases of meningitis tuberculosa, miliary tubercles of the pharyngeal
mucosa that are unattended by subjective symptoms.

I have seen one case in which destruction of the
soft palate, with subsequent extension to the pillars
and tonsils, resulted from ulceration of the floor of the
nose and upper surface of the palate.

Age: The disease does not show any limitations in
the age extremes of those attacked but the majority of
the cases occur in the period between and including
puberty and late adolescence. Although neither extreme of age is exempt, the condition is much more frequently met with in the very young than in those of advanced years.

V. Santvoord (Tuberculosis of the Lungs, &c., New
York Medical Record, March 14, 1885) records a case
occurring in an infant of 18 months, and reference has
already been made to Isambert's case of primary pharyngitis in a boy of four and one-half years. All of
Abercrombies' three cases (On three Cases of Ac. Tuberc. Ulc. of Fauces, British Med. Journal, Nov. 13,
1886) occurred in young children, and P. Schötz
(*Deutsche medicinische Wochenschrift*, Oct. 15, 1903)
saw two cases in children of eight and ten years of age.

Of 35 cases assembled by Barth, two were over 60

years of age. The great majority have occurred between the years of 20 and 35.

In the author's series of 39 cases there was but one under 20 years, a boy of 11 with widespread involvement of the pillars and posterior wall, and only one was over 36 years, a woman of 47. Nearly all occurred between the ages of 22 and 30, and in all the process was secondary to disease of the lungs, or lungs and other organs.

Sex: Pharyngeal tuberculosis is much more common in males than in females, the disproportion being considerably greater than in laryngeal tuberculosis and almost the exact opposite of what obtains in the nose. A study of all available reports gives an approximate proportion of four to one. There seems to be no adequate explanation of this greater vulnerability on the part of the male, and it bears no relation to the frequency with which the two sexes are attacked by pulmonary phthisis. Twenty-eight of the thirty-nine patients seen by the author were men.

Esophagus: It has been seen that in the respiratory tract the tuberculous infections decrease markedly in frequency as we ascend from the lungs to the external openings, but in the upper alimentary tract the exact converse obtains and the esophagus occupies somewhat the same position as the nose.

Up to the year 1898, Cone (*Münchener medicinishe Wochenschr., Nr. 5, 1898*) was able to assemble but 48 cases and only a few additional ones have been since reported. The reason for this infrequency is readily seen when the conformation of the tube and its physiological functions are studied.

the smooth walls are quickly washed away by the passing food and drink.

That these are the main protective agencies is witnessed by the fact that a primary infection of the esophagus is practically unknown;—nearly all recorded cases have occurred as the result of direct extension from contiguous tissues.

In a few instances the tuberculous process has been grafted upon a pre-existing lesion, such as syphilis, carcinoma or traumatic ulcers. Abrasions of the mucosa, be their character what they may, offer a favorable nidus for the development of the bacilli, but a primary infection of the uninjured tube has so far not been observed.

PLATE XXIV.

Fig. 76. Ulceration of the esophagus secondary to extensive disease of the larynx.

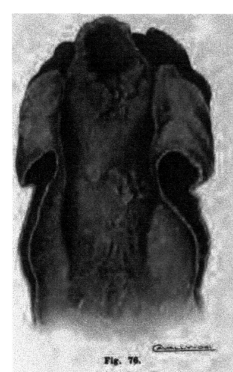

Fig. 76.

In a patient who had drunk caustic potash and had in consequence many cicatrices of the esophagus, Breus (*Tuberculöse Ulcer. des Pharynx, Oesophagus und Magens nach Kalilaugenätzung, Wiener. Med. Wochenschr., Nr.* II, 1878) found at autopsy a number of tuberculous ulcers in the pharynx, esophagus and stomach, and Kundrat (*Wiener med. Wochenschr.* Bd. XXXIV, Nos. 6 & 7, 1884) saw a similar case due to the drinking of sulphuric acid.

Zemann (*Tuberculose des Oesophagus, Anz. d. Ges. d. Ae. in Wien,* No. 31, 1886) saw one case of a like nature, while Eppinger (*Ueb. Tuberculose des Magens und des Oesophagus, Prager med. Wochenschrift,* Nos. 51 & 52, 1881) observed a woman in whom miliary tubercles and ulcers were found throughout the entire extent of the esophagus, which before cleansing had been almost entirely occluded by mould.

The development of tuberculosis upon a carcinomatous base has been described by a number of observers, i. e., Lubarsch, Pepper, Edsall, Zenker, and Cordua.

Beck and Zenker have reported cases in which the esophageal ulceration advanced subepithelially from the pharyngo-laryngeal portion of the gullet, and Mazzotti (*Delle alterazioni dell esofago nella tuberculosi, Rivista Clinica,* 1, 1885) had two cases in which the esophageal ulcers were associated with intestinal tuberculosis. In one case there were some simple denudations of the gullet through which infection undoubtedly occurred.

Mazzoti observed another case, a boy of 10 years, who had a caseating bronchial gland and general miliary tuberculosis.

quent perforation and extension of the process beneath or in the epithelium.

Bartlett (*Ann. Otol. Rhin. and Laryngol.*, Nov., 1899) reports two such cases; in one there was one fistula, in the other five, leading to as many different peribronchial and posterior mediastinal glands.

While such a perforation almost always results in a spread of the disease to the lining of the tube, the process sometimes stops at this point and the perforation may close spontaneously. Cases of perforation without esophageal foci are recorded by Penrose, Neumann, Poland, Nowak, Barry, Hanot, and Völcker.

The condition often runs a symptomless course and it is probably due to this factor, as well as to the difficulty of diagnosis during life, that such a small number of cases are recorded.

Faucial Tonsils: The study of tonsillar tuberculosis may be said to date from the thesis of Dieulafoy entitled, "Latent Tuberculosis of the Three Tonsils," (1895) in which he reported the results of numerous inoculations of guinea pigs with portions of hyperplastic tonsils and adenoid vegetations taken from individuals presumably non-tuberculous, and from which he drew the following conclusions:

"There is another form of tuberculosis of the Palato-nasopharynx which is much more frequent. If this form to which I allude has for a long time passed unperceived, it is because it does not correspond to any of the forms of pharyngeal tubercle just sketched. This form is neither ulcerous nor granular; it is not at all painful; it remains unknown until the day when it reveals itself by certain functional troubles; it is benign in appearance, but is none the less formidable, for it is sometimes the portal of entrance of a generalized tuberculosis and of pulmonary phthisis.

"This tuberculosis is torpid, concealed, almost latent, having as its favorite seat the lymphoid tissue of the naso-pharynx. It reveals itself by a greater or less enlargement of this tissue, by a hypertrophy of one or more of the tonsillar structures. As concerns the pharyngeal tonsil, it confounds itself with the condition known as adenoid vegetations; as concerns the faucial tonsils, with the condition known as simple hypertrophy. Inspection in no wise reveals the nature of the lesion. It does not present, I repeat, on inspection,

(1.) In thirty-four consecutive post-mortems, the tonsils were found tuberculous in twenty. In the majority of the cases the tonsils were atrophied; in two there was slight hypertrophy and in none had there been any subjective symptoms referable to the throat.

(2). All examinations negative.

Other observers, however, have found primary tonsillar tubercles in a considerable percentage of their cases. Ruge, in 18 cases, found definite signs of tuberculosis in six.

Baup gives a table of 841 tonsils examined by different investigators, of which 53 (or about six per cent) showed tuberculous involvement.

Rethi (*Wiener Klin. Rundschau*, July 1, 1900) found

bacilli in six of 100 hypertrophied tonsils taken from subjects showing no signs of tuberculosis.

Von Schreiber (*Deutsche Med. Wochenschr.*, May 25, 1889) examined a large number of tonsils taken from apparently sound indiivduals and found tubercles in three.

C. M. Robertson (Journal American Med. Assoc., Nov. 24, 1906) found 8 per cent of 232 tonsils, removed from living patients, to be tuberculous.

G. B. Wood (Journ. Amer. Med. Assoc., May 6, 1905) concludes, from his investigations and the published records of 1671 cases of hypertrophied tonsils, that at least 5 per cent of all hypertrophied pharyngeal tonsils conceal latent tuberculous lesions, but that the faucial tonsils are more rarely involved.

In individuals with tuberculosis of other organs tonsillar involvements are the rule. In addition to the figures already cited we have the statistics of Strassmann and Krückmann.

The former found the tonsils affected in fifteen of twenty-one cases examined, and the latter twelve times in twelve cases of cervical lymphadenitis, and in forty-eight of fifty cases of advanced phthisis. In thirty-four cases of moderate pulmonary involvement they were affected in only six.

Schlenker found eight cases of bilateral tonsillar involvement, and one of unilateral, in nine consumptives having advanced disease. In nine other cases, with only moderate pulmonary involvement, the tonsils were affected in two, and in five children with either mild or only moderately advanced disease of the lungs, the tonsils were tuberculous in three.

there is a formation, not only of lymphoid tissue but of actual crypts and follicles as well.

Sokolowski examined the granular tissue of the pharynx and lateral folds of 13 consumptives and found latent tubercles in eight, or 61 1-2 per cent of the cases.

The lingual tonsil was found to be tuberculous in nine of fifteen consumptives examined by Dmochowski.

In these cases of secondary infection the bacillus must have been deposited by the sputum in the majority of cases, in others by the blood or lymphatic current. but in those in whom the disease is localized in the tonsil. infection occurs through primary deposit at this point by the air or ingesta.

Schlesinger (*D. Tubercul. d. Tonsillen. b. Kindern. Berl. Klinik.* 99, 1896) records a case in which the infection travelled, via the lymphatics, from a focus in the petrous portion of the temporal bone to the cervical glands, and from them to the tonsils.

Retrograde infection from the cervical glands has been proven in a considerable number of cases.

Since the bacillus is known to pass through intact mucous membranes without necessarily leaving trace of its passage, and can pass on into other and more vulnerable tissues, the tonsils, in view of the considerable percentage of cases in which tubercles are found without other demonstrable foci, assume considerable importance as a portal through which infections gain a foothold.

A direct connection between these tonsillar infections and cervical adenitis has been shown in a large series of cases. From his own investigations and a review of the literature, Walsham concludes:

(1.) That the tonsils, instead of being almost immune from tuberculous disease, are very frequently affected.

(2). That tubercle may be primary in the tonsil.

(3). That the tonsils are very frequently affected secondarily in persons suffering with chronic tuberculosis.

(4). That when the tonsils are tuberculous, the cervical glands receiving the lymphatics from these organs are also frequently affected with tubercle.

(5). That the follicular glands at the base of the tongue are occasionally found tuberculous.

(6). That tonsils may be affected from without or through the blood stream in acute miliary tuberculosis.

The conditions favoring the entrance of the bacilli into the tonsils, their retention and development, have been shown on pages 311 and 313, so these factors, holding true in respect to the faucial lymphoid tissue as well, need not be reiterated. There remain to be quoted only some additional facts regarding the part this tissue plays in the further dissemination of the disease.

Tuberculosis may develop at any point and in any apices.

This source of infection has been carefully investigated by different observers with different results and conclusions.

Grogler injected the tonsils of living animals with India ink and was able to demonstrate its passage, via the lymphatics, into the pleural apices and bronchial glands. From the case reports of various observers he also found that 14.3 per cent of patients with tuberculous cervical lymphadenitis developed tuberculosis of the pleura.

Beitzke attacked these experiments after extensive anatomical and experimental studies, and summarized as follows:

"(1). There exist no lymph vessels leading from the chain of cervical lymph glands to the bronchial glands.

"(2). Tuberculous infiltration of the lungs from cervical lymph glands can take place only through the lymphatic trunk and the venous system.

"(3). This path of infection, at least in children, is without any practical import. The infection of the lungs, and hence the bronchial glands, in children as a rule takes place through aspiration of the tubercle bacillus into the bronchi; a descending tuberculosis may be present incidentally.

"(4). The aspirated bacilli may be in the respired air but they come from the mouth where they may have gained access by food or by contact."

Wood's experiments support Beitzke's claim concerning the connection between the supraclavicular lymph glands and those higher up in the neck but, on the other hand, he showed that:

"In children the number and arrangement is very irregular, and that the pleural apices come into fairly close relation not only with the supraclavicular glands but also with the extreme lower portion of the greater vessels of the neck.

"The deep lateral chain of the neck extends downward along these vessels, and if there should be a node situated in the lower part of the neck, as sometimes occurs, it is conceivable that the tuberculosis of this node may infect the pleural apices directly by continuity of structure."

In a previous chapter it has been shown that laryngeal infection in some cases has its apparent origin in a glandular focus.

Inoculation experiments by Cornet show how generalized infections sometimes result from induced foci in the tonsils, posterior pharyngeal wall, and mouth.

Seven animals were inoculated in the lateral pockets of the mouth, two in the tonsils, two in the tongue, and two in the posterior pharynx. In every case there ensued cheesy degeneration of the submental, sublingual and cervical glands, and in some instances nodules appeared in the lungs, and later on in the spleen. An ulcer generally occurred, after about three weeks, at the point of inoculation, although in some instances no local changes were observable.

A clinical case of great interest in this connection is recorded by Koplik (Amer. Journal Med. Sciences, Nov., 1903). A child who had died of acute general miliary tuberculosis showed on autopsy that the only old cheesy foci were located in the tonsil, strong evidence that the disease had originated at that point.

Walsham refers to a number of somewhat parallel cases, in which all the post-mortem evidence pointed to lesions of the tonsils as the foci of dissemination.

While we as yet have little data of definite value concerning the influence of the tonsils and glands in causing generalized tuberculosis, all the work that has been done points to the fact that they are of considerable etiologic importance.

The latent foci show slight tendency to destruction or cheesy degeneration, although ulceration does exceptionally result. As a rule they gradually disappear

PLATE XXV.

Fig. 77. Edema of the pillars of the tonsils, with small group of incipient tubercules on the soft palate

Fig. 77. Infiltration and edema of the pillars of the tonsils.

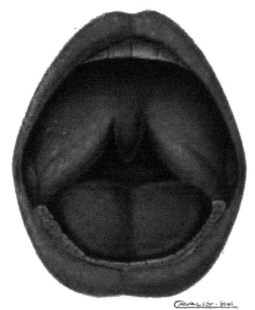

Fig, 77.

PLATE XXV.

FIG. 77.   Infiltration and edema of the pillars of the tonsils.

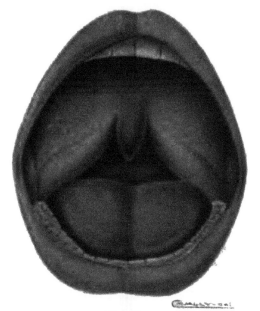

Fig. 77.

PLATE

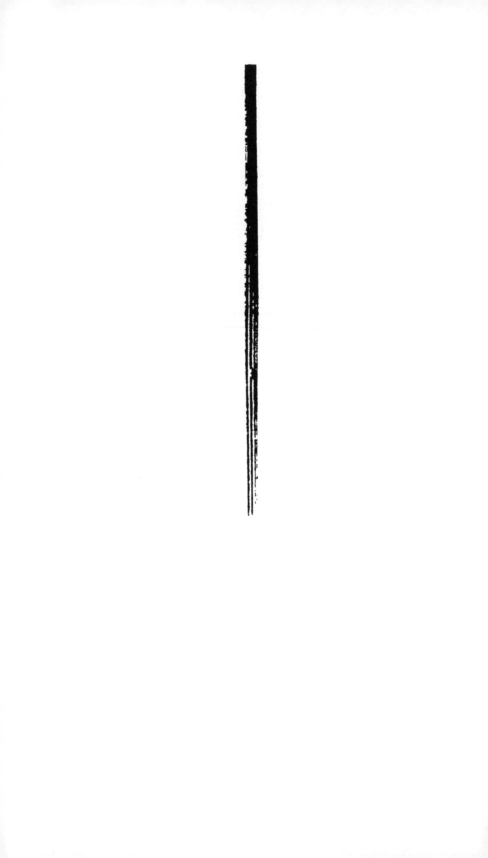

through the process of retrograde metamorphosis which is a characteristic of all tonsillar tissue.

Apparently primary tuberculosis of the tonsils, of an ulcerative type, has been observed in a considerable number of instances. The two cases recorded by Orth and Kürckmann in which the condition was present in children suffering from diphtheria, have already been mentioned.

Abraham (Dublin Journal of Med. Science, Oct., 1885) recorded a case of tonsillar ulceration occurring in a woman in whom there were no other demonstrable foci, and Ruge observed a like condition in an eighteen year old girl otherwise normal.

In Lennox Browne's case, prevously referred to, there was tuberculous ulceration of the left tonsil but neither the lungs nor larynx was affected. Ozeki (*Internat. Centralb. f. Laryn.*, Sept., 1900) reports two personal cases.

A number of other isolated cases are on record.

SYMPTOMS.

Subjective: Latent tonsillar tuberculosis presents no subjective symptoms, and when ulceration has occurred the manifestations are identical _with those evoked by a breaking down of the other segments of the pharynx, hence the clinical picture may be presented without an attempt to consider each segment by itself.

The one, great, predominant symptom of pharyngeal tuberculosis is pain. In the very early days of the outbreak there may be nothing more than a sensation of tickling, of constriction, or as of a foreign body, but this rapidly changes to one of actual pain, unremitting. and severe, with extreme exacerbations upon all attempts at swallowing food or mucus, and upon use of the voice. Great quantities of mucus are poured out which, thick and tenacious in character, add greatly to the sufferer's discomfort. The pain is greatest in the pharynx but extends in lancinating attacks to the ears by transference through the nerves, i. e., the vagus and glossopharyngeus and its tympanic branch, Jacobson's nerve.

The pain increases rapidly until, generally within a comparatively few days, it becomes so severe that the patient voluntarily abstains from all food and drink, preferring starvation to the agony attendant upon swallowing. Lesions of the palate may, exceptionally, run an almost painless course and I have seen one case of pharyngeal ulceration that occasioned nothing more than moderate discomfort.

Regurgitation of food, both liquid and solid, is an almost invariable result of advanced disease, because of the imperfect closure of the naso-pharynx by the palate.

This failure of the palate to perform its functions gives to the voice a hard, so-called "palatal" quality, closely resembling that so characteristic of other painful affections of the tonsils and pillars, i. e., peritonsillar abscess, plegmon, &c.

The temperature is usually somewhat elevated and there is rapid loss of strength and weight, with a general increase of activity in all other existing foci.

The pyrexia is due not so much to the pharynx itself as to the accompanying disease of the lungs or other in-

PLATE XXVI.

Fig. 78. General ulceration of the palate, extending forward upon the hard palate. Uvula infiltrated, with crenated borders.

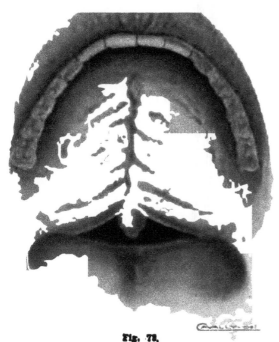

Fig. 78.

PLATE XXVI.

fected organs, which is always more or less aggravated by the malnutrition, pain, cough and restlessness consequent upon the pharyngeal outbreak.

In primary infections of the pharynx the temperature is rarely elevated to any great extent, although it may rise one or two degrees.

Several severe cases have been noted in which no increase whatsoever occurred, but, on the other hand, hyperpyrexia has occurred in a number of instances.

Mackenzie had one case in which the temperature ranged as high as 104 degrees, and upon one occasion rose to 106 degrees.

In one of Fränkel's cases the temperature curve resembled that of typhoid and in another it rose to 107.06 degrees.

The breath is invariably foul but this is undoubtedly due, in large part, to the accompanying pulmonic disease.

OBJECTIVE SYMPTOMS.

The macroscopic images in pharyngeal tuberculosis are usually quite characteristic, for by the time the subjective symptoms are sufficiently pronounced to direct attention to the throat, the process has usually advanced so far that no doubt as to the diagnosis can arise.

The process is generally so fulminant that little opportunity is afforded of studying the condition in its incipient stages (congestion and circumscribed infiltration) such as we see in the larynx, and we have to deal, as a rule, with an already widespread ulceration or advanced tubercle or miliary formation.

Uncomplicated diffuse infiltration is the rarest of all forms and seldom comes to observation, owing to the fact that the parts are subject to almost constant motion and the thermic and chemical irritation by the ingesta and secretions, with consequent ulceration at a very early period.

The infiltrate tends to spread more deeply into the tissue than in other parts, and because of the almost constant presence of some edema, is more transparent and colorless in appearance.

The most vulnerable points are the pillars of the tonsils and in these localities the edematous infiltration may be so great as to produce enormous thickening, sufficient at times to absolutely destroy the normal contour of the pharynx.

They become gelatinous in appearance, are markedly convex in both diameters, and may be covered by either a smooth or warty mucosa which contains numerous submucous miliary nodules. Such a case is shown in Plate XXV., Fig. 77.

This patient, a man of 35, had had both pulmonary and laryngeal tuberculosis for about one year when the palatal infiltration appeared. The condition in both the lungs and larynx was rapidly nearing the stage of arrest, when he developed some dysphagia and odynophagia. The posterior pillars of both tonsils were found to be enormously infiltrated, making contact with the anterior folds and completely hiding the underlying tonsils.

The uvula was congested but not edematous, and on the right side the soft palate, immediately above the anterior pillar, showed several incipient miliary

PLATE XXVII.

FIG. 79. Ulceration of the tonsil involving the anterior and posterior pillars, showing characteristic profuse granulation tissue.

Fig. 79.

PLATE XXVII.

tubercles. The swellings had a transparent, gelatinous appearance, and the mucosa was smooth and glistening.

Within a few days the entire mass broke down and became covered with innumerable spots of ulceration, varying in size from a pinpoint to an almond seed, and in less than two weeks the process had extended over the entire soft palate and uvula.

This condition is shown in Plate XXVI., Fig. 78, made fifteen days after the preceding illustration.

In some rare cases the entire soft palate, uvula and pillars are infiltrated to such an extent that they become board-like in consistency, dense, firm, rigid and unyielding.

At the present time the writer has a patient under observation in whom all of these structures are so infiltrated that they are absolutely immobile. The soft palate is extensively ulcerated, but neither the uvula nor pillars have as yet given way to the constantly increasing pressure of the infiltrate, and yet the tip of the uvula can scarcely be moved, and the swollen tissues encroach so much upon the pharyngeal aperture that there is not sufficient space for the introduction of the smallest mirror.

In the more common form of the disease we see a swollen and more or less anemic mucous membrane, through the surface of which glisten numerous small gray or yellow tubercles. The mucosa surrounding these groups may be slightly inflamed, although as a rule it has a pale and lifeless appearance.

The tubercles rapidly disintegrate and form superfiscal ulcers within a period of a few days to two or three weeks. These are absolutely pathognomonic and their favored sites are the soft palate and the uvula, and then the tonsils and posterior wall.

The resultant ulcers are lenticular in form and extend toward the periphery rather than into the deeper structures; the edges are irregular, "mouse" · or "worm" eaten, and merge gradually into normal tissue, although they may occasionally be slightly infiltrated or undermined. An areole of moderate hyperemia may or may not be present.

The infiltration is generally so slight as to be scarcely appreciable, and the floor is dotted with minute palered granulations which are commonly obscured by a tenacious dirty yellow secretion. These are especially profuse upon the tonsils and posterior wall. (Plate XXVII., Fig. 79).

In some instances the ulcers are covered by a deposit that bears a strong resemblance to the membrane formed in diphtheria, and when this becomes confluent and covers large areas of the tonsils and posterior wall, it may give rise to some difficulties in diagnoss, especially as in this type there is high fever, severe pain, prostraton, and occasionally some dyspnea.

In the immediate vicinity of the ulcer minute miliary tubercles usually appear, which soon disintegrate, causing rapid extension to all contiguous parts.

The occurrence of a true miliary tuberculosis of the pharynx is extremely rare, and as a rule is a manifestation of a general miliary tuberculosis but the pharynx is occasionally the only site of the disease.

I have seen two cases in which the outbreak occurred

PLATE XXVIII.

FIG. 80. Extensive tuberculous ulceration of the pharynx, pillars, uvula and palate.

palate.

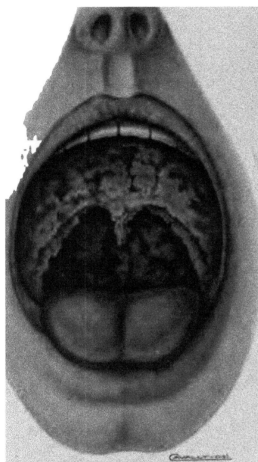

Fig. 80.

PLATE XXVIII.

in association with a miliary laryngitis. One of these recovered, the other died within two months.

Other cases have been described by Löri, Cadier, Küer, Rethi, Catti, Letulle, Fränkel, and a few other observers.

On the posterior walls the ulcers may be round, oval or irregular, but occasionally they assume a pronounced stellate form. When the tonsil is extensively involved, large portions of the organ may melt away with great rapidity; at certain points the ulceration extends to the basal membrane, while the tissue in the intermediate spaces is so friable and granular that it can be torn away, piece by piece, with the greatest ease. In these cases the tonsil appears as though it were the seat of a virulent gangrene, and severe bleeding may occur. Ordinarily the tuberculous process is not productive of hemorrhages, and in the case reported by Fränkel in which there was much bleeding the tuberculosis was complicated by a mercurial stomatitis.

The uvula is frequently affected at an early stage of the disease. It may be thickened to from two to five times its normal size by a collection of numerous, hard, wart-like tubercles, giving it the so-called "thumb" shape. In other cases small yellow miliary tubercles or minute ulcers, resembling the spots produced in herpes after the breaking down of the vesicles, dot its entire surface.

In time many of the various areas become confluent and the throat appears as though it were covered by one immense ulcer or adherent membrane, that extends in some instances into the naso-pharynx, in others to the tongue and larynx, or the cheeks and gums. (Plate XXVIII, Fig. 80.)

Death usually intervenes before there is time for much actual loss of tissue—except in cases of tonsillar ulceration—but sometimes a large part of the palate or uvula disappears.

Cicatricial bands between the palate and posterior pharyngeal wall, such as are seen after syphilitic disease, rarely form, owing to the failure of any permanent reparative efforts. Kraus, however, (*Nothnagel's Handbuch*, XVI, I, Th. 1, Abth., p. 276) reports several such cases.

Perforations of the palate have been observed in a small number of instances and are of especial importance because of the likelihood of their being confused with syphilis.

Comparatively few such cases have been recorded and these embrace lesions of both the hard and soft palate.

Ulceration not leading to perforation, on the other hand, is fairly frequent, and in a few well authenticated cases seem to have been the primary localization of the disease. (Plate XXIX., Fig. 81).

Küssner saw four such cases, one was reported by Kessler, and one by Uckermann. This last case (Uckermann's) was completely cured.

According to Guttmann, nearly one per cent of the cases of phthisis seen by him had tuberculous ulceration of the palate and soft palate, and of the 114 cases of local tuberculosis reported by Delavan (New York Med. Jour., May 14, 1887) 8 had ulceration of the velum.

PLATE XXIX.

Fig. 81. Circumscribed ulceration of the soft palate.

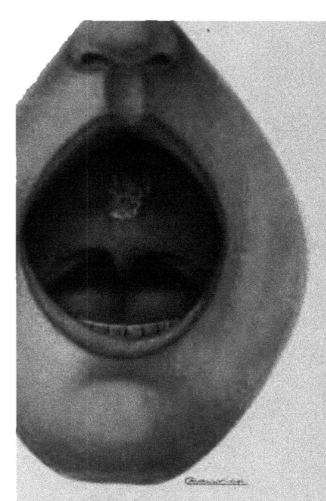

Fig. 81.

PLATE XXIX.

Wagner saw two patients with tuberculosis of the soft palate, both of whom had had syphilis, and Aguanno saw tuberculosis become grafted upon a specific ulcer of the velum.

Newcomb, in 1904 (Tuberculosis of the Pharynx, Laryngoscope, June, 1904), was able to find but 11 cases in which perforation had occurred, 10 of which had been assembled by Grogler. Of these ten cases, eight occurred in patients with well marked disease of the lungs or larynx.

In one case of Kayser's (*Monatschr. f. Ohrenheilk.*, 8-9, 1905) the perforation affected the left anterior palatine arch, and one case is recorded in which necrosis of the hard palate resulted, necessitating extensive removal of the bone.

Barbier (Journ. Laryn., London, April 2, 1899) saw one case of perforation of the soft palate that followed a severe attack of influenza.

The process is extremely sluggish, and examination reveals an inflammatory areola enclosing a bloody and purulent ulcer, dotted here and there by numerous pale or red granulations. The borders are irregular, superficial and mouse-eaten. The ulcer gradually increases in depth without much lateral spread, until perforation results.

The opening is sinuous in form and lies at the bottom of a deep and irregular fissure or cleft, and is always solitary.

Aside from these acute and sub-acute lesions, due to direct infection of the pharyngeal tissues, there is in addition an essentially chronic process in which the posterior pharynx is involved by extension from a neighboring focus in the vertebral column. This appears in the pharynx as a cold abscess, and the symptoms are those due to the vertebral disease associated with a large fluctuating tumor in the retropharynx, the location of which depends upon the particular verterba affected. In very young children the abscess is generally confined to one side—a central localization is extremely rare—and it may be located either high up behind the velum palati or low down in the pharynx.

The symptoms, as a rule, are insidious.

There is little attendant inflammation and attention is generally first drawn to the throat by the development of dysphagia and dyspnea. The voice has a palatal quality, the so-called "Crie de Canard" of Reigenier, and there is a hacking cough. There may or may not be pain but there is always some tenderness on pressure.

Adenitis of the cervical and sub-maxillary glands may occur in all forms of pharyngeal tuberculosis, but even the severer types may be unaccompanied by any signs of enlargement or sensitiveness. It may occur either early or late in the course of the disease, the degree of pharyngeal involvement seemingly bearing no relation to the frequency of glandular infections.

Tuberculomata do not occur in the pharynx; at least they have not as yet been observed, although Avellis (*Deutsche med. Wochensch.*, Nr. 32 and 33, 1891) describes their occurrence on the posterior surface of the uvula.

Masses of granulation tissue resembling tuberculomata have occurred upon the tonsils and uvula, and in the case of Schnitzler's, already described, the in

PLATE XXX.

FIG. 82. Triple perforation of the soft palate and anterior pillar of syphilitic origin, in a patient with pulmonary tuberculosis (Case seen by courtesy of Dr. D. S. Newman).

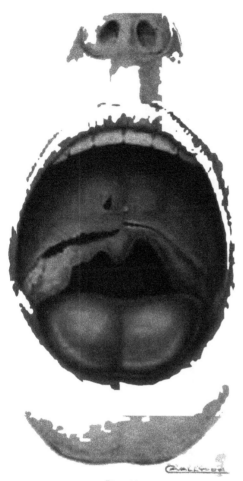

Fig. 82.

PLATE XXX.

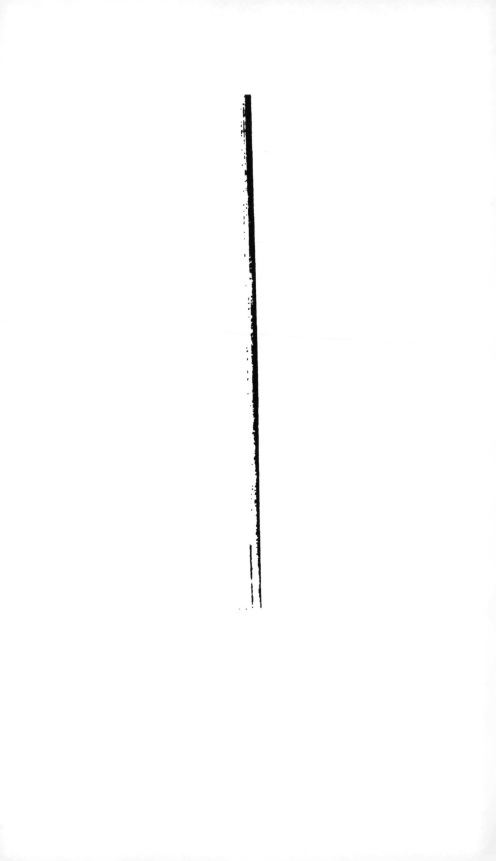

jection of tuberculin caused the eruption of numerous miliary tubercles that became aggregated in tumor-like masses upon the posterior pharyngeal wall and within the naso-pharynx. These, however, are not instances of true tuberculomata, which, in the strict meaning of the term, are tumor-like growths not preceded nor accompanied by ulceration.

DIAGNOSIS.

A tuberculous lesion of the pharynx is so characteristic in appearance that, once seen, it can scarcely be mistaken for any other condition.

Certain of the rarer types, however, and atypical forms of the more common varieties may give rise to some temporary confusion.

First in the list of diseases with which it may be confused is syphilis. In their typical manifestations no points of similarity exist; the lesions of both are pathogonomonic, and the extra-laryngeal symptoms are so constant and clear that a mistake in differentiation is rarely possible. The classical features of each are pictured on page 132.

When doubts do arise, the therapeutic test and microscopic examination of scrapings from the ulcerated spots will soon show their true nature.

Herpes may sometimes closely simulate tuberculosis, and particularly when occurring in phthisical individuals. The herpetic eruption in the beginning consists of numerous small vesicles that are not easily mistaken, but when these break down into ulcers and become covered by a yellowish false membrane, they may bear a striking similarity to miliary tubercles.

They appear upon all parts of the pharynx, the posterior wall, pillars, tonsils and palate, and are accompanied by severe pain, odynophagia and muffling of the voice. Herpes runs an acute course, however, and this clears the diagnosis within a few days.

Thrush likewise may be confused with an acute miliary outbreak in the pharynx, but the patches of membrane are easily detached and under the microscope show the oidium albicans. In both of these diseases the areas of mucosa between the spots are much more hyperemic than in tuberculosis.

Between lupus and tuberculosis we have, in the former condition, an afebrile course, sensitiveness rather than pain, complete absence of dysphagia and odynophagia, a sluggish development, and points of ulceration, tubercle formation, and cicatrization side by side. Tuberculosis shows no tendency towards spontaneous healing, hence scar tissue is never present.

When palatal ulceration has advanced to perforation, a number of conditions must be taken into consideration: trauma, syphilis, malignancy, the Mal Perforant Buccal, and openings of a congenital origin.

The perforation due to syphilis is generally of large size, has a distinct, punched-out appearance, has no contiguous yellow granulations, and is usually provocative of more extensive necrosis than the opening due to tuberculosis, and other signs of the disease can practically always be uncovered. (Plate XXX., Fig. 82).

In tuberculosis sequestra never form and there is never more than one opening; in syphilis there may be several, and the former condition attacks by prefer-

PLATE XXXI.

FIG. 83. A deep linear tuberculous ulcer of the tongue; the sharply circumscribed infiltrate, the undermined edges and deep extension give an image more typical of syphilis than of tuberculosis.

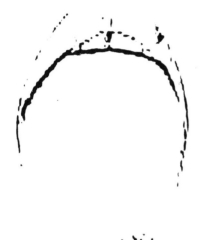

Fig. 82.

PLATE XXXI.

ence the middle part of the velum, while syphilis usually affects the osseous walls.

The mucosa in syphilis is red and angry, in tuberculosis generally anemic.

In tuberculosis, the pharyngeal process is frequently associated with characteristic lesions of the gums, lips and tongue. (Fig. 70, Plate XIX., Fig. 83, Plate XXXI., Fig. 84, Plate XXXII., and Fig. 85, Plate XXXII.)

The Mal Perforant Buccal, according to Newcomb, has been noted especially in tabes, and may follow pyorrhea alveolaris. He says:

"In the tabetic cases, we find sensory disturbances in the trigeminal area, especially close to the ulceration. The openings are often bilaterally symmetrical, and occur by preference at the periphery of the bone near the alveolar border, in a direction parallel to the axis of which the ulcer is elongated. The openings are of considerable size, and the attempts at repair are indolent."

PROGNOSIS.

The prognosis in both the primary and secondary forms of the disease is usually unfavorable. Lesions of an incipient character may occasionally be overcome, but when they have once gained a firm foothold, especially if associated with severe pulmonary or laryngeal phthisis, one is not justified in holding out any hope of arrest or even temporary betterment.

Treatment for the purpose of local palliation and of producing euthanasia, is almost equally futile. Occasionally, when the infected areas are strictly circumscribed or even when widely distributed, if shallow and non-confluent, arrest may ensue. Such cases, however, are of the greatest rarity.

The lesions limited to the posterior wall offer the best chance of arrest.

Gleitsmann reports one case of primary tuberculosis of the mouth and pharynx in which a cure was attained, and Theisen (Jour. Amer. Med. Assoc., Aug. 12, 1899) cured one case in which both the lungs and larynx were involved in addition to the pharynx.

I have seen two cases with a favorable issue: one, a patient with an acute miliary outbreak in the larynx and pharynx (Case X, page 132) recovered and was living eighteen months after the last symptoms disappeared; the other has made a partial recovery, but only two months have elapsed since the last vestige of ulceration disappeared and there is still considerable infiltration of the posterior pillars. During the pharyngeal outbreak there was recurrence in the larynx, and the epiglottis, previously unaffected, became involved.

This case can naturally be classed only under the head of "temporary improvement."

The remaining 37 patients all died within from two to fifteen weeks from the onset of the disease, and in all the pharyngeal process was complicated by advanced disease of both the lungs and larynx.

Veis (Arch. f. Laryng., XII, 1902) reports a few cases cured by trichloracetic acid. Isolated cases of a like nature have been reported by various observers, i. e., one case each by

Boluminski (Beitr. z. Tuberc. d. ob. Luftwege, Diss. erlangen, 1895);

PLATE XXXII.

FIG. 84. Extensive tuberculous ulcer of the lip in a patient with advanced disease of the lungs and larynx.

FIG. 85. Tuberculous ulcer of the tongue (Dr. T. E. Carmody).

Fig.   Tuberculous ulcer of the tongue.

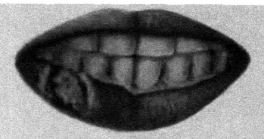

Fig. 84.

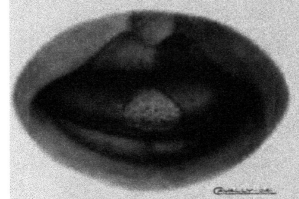

Fig. 85.

PLATE X

Schmiegelow (*Hospitals-Tidende* 49, 1884);

Seifert (*Handbuch der. Laryn. u. Rhinologie*, pg. 730);

Luc (*Arch. d. lar.*, Nr. 1, 1889);

Wróblewski (*Wien med. Pr.*, 14, 1893);

Pluder (*Deutsche med. Wochenschr. Vereinsbeil*, 6, 1896);

Doutrelepont (*Deutsche med. Wochenschr.*, 46, 1892);

Heryng (*Gaz. lek.* 31, 1892);

Talamon (*Ann. d. mal. d l'Or.*, *Nr.* 5, 1894);

Uckermann (*Norsk. Magaz. f. Laegevidensk.*, 1884); and Finkler (*Berl. Klin. Wochenschr.*, 1884.)

Each of the following has seen two cases of healing:

Lennox Browne (*Centralbl. f. Laryngologie*, IV, 1888);

Küssner (*Deutsche med. Wochenschr.*, 1881).

Additional cures are reported by Michelson (*Deutsche med. Wochenschr.*, pg. 718, 1891); Renvers (*Deutsche med. Wochenschr.*, 14, 1891); Rosenberg (*D. Krankh. d. Mundhöhle*, 1893), and Carmody (personal report).

The proportion of cures to the total number of cases, however, is so small that one is scarcely justified in anticipating anything but rapid and uninterrupted progression, with death within a comparatively few weeks.

Isolated disease of the tonsils, either secondary or latent, may be completely cured if the entire organ is promptly and thoroughly extirpated, although the traumatism is sometimes accountable for the accession of pulmonary phthisis.

When palatal perforations occur, independent of any other local or general focus, they sometimes close spontaneously; if they are of considerable size, they may be permanently repaired by operation.

TREATMENT.

The treatment of tuberculous pharyngitis falls naturally into two divisions: curative and palliative.

· The former should embrace, primarily at the least, all cases in which the lesions are fairly circumscribed, and particularly if limited to the posterior wall or tonsil, regardless of the state of the lungs and larynx.

The reason for this is plain: the process, if unchecked, leads invariably to excruciating and unconquerable pain, and hence every effort should be put forth to cause cicatrization, even when the general disease is so far advanced as to render the prospect of cure or even temporary arrest absolutely hopeless.

The same effort is justifiable in extensive pharyngeal disease unassociated with other lesions that would of themselves prove fatal. If, however, radical intervention is made in cases combining advanced pharyngeal and pulmonary or laryngeal tuberculosis, where the general vitality is low, harm only can result, for new and increased activity is the rule in such cases, and the suffering of the unfortunate patient is more apt to be aggravated than lessend.

Radical or curative treatment consists in the use of the curette, electric or thermo-cautery, and cauterizing pigments, of which the most effective are formalin and lactic acid. All of these agents have been minutely considered in the chapter on treatment of laryngeal tuberculosis, and since the same general principles apply to the pharynx as to other segments of the throat, no separate description is required.

Palliative Treatment: Palliative treatment is much less effective than in the larynx. In the latter location a radical removal of the affected tissues is frequently possible, but in the pharynx such a procedure is only rarely advisable.

Likewise, the various medicaments brought into contact with the laryngeal mucosa can be retained for a considerable period, while in the pharynx they are almost immediately removed by the constant motion to which the parts are subjected by the passing secretions, the muscular contractures during deglutition, &c.

The powders, for this reason, are largely without effect, and because of their drying properties are extremely disagreeable. Neither can we make use of the oily preparations holding the anesthetic powders in solution, which, upon evaporation, leave a film of powder over the affected spots.

In fact, we are reduced largely to the use of one class of remedies, the local anesthetics, cocain, alypin, &c.

The patient should be permitted to use these *ad libitum*, in gradually increasing strengths, with occasional interchange from one to the other, in order to avoid in so far as possible the development of a more or less pronounced toleration. Orthoform and anesthesin, insufflated thoroughly upon the ulcerated spots, will give some fleeting relief and may be used in connection with other remedies.

Curettement, with the after application of one of the cauterizing pigments, oftimes affords some relief.

INDEX

.

Lightning Source UK Ltd.
Milton Keynes UK
UKHW012252110219
337137UK00006B/875/P